David A. Dosser, Jr., PhD
Dorothea Handron, EdD
Susan McCammon, PhD
John Y. Powell, PhD
Editors

Child Mental Health: Exploring Systems of Care in the New Millennium

Child Mental Health: Exploring Systems of Care in the New Millennium has been co-published simultaneously as *Journal of Family Social Work*, Volume 5, Number 3 2001.

Pre-publication REVIEWS, COMMENTARIES, EVALUATIONS . . .

"At last, a book about training personnel for human services work that puts the rhetoric of systems of care into action! This book will guide changes in the way universities train human services personnel. Individual chapters detail specific instructional strategies for conveying the model and applying it by developing new kinds of professional skills. Readily understandable by family members and across the human services disciplines."

Trina W. Osher, MA
Coordinator
Policy & Research
Federation of Families for Children's Mental Health
Tacoma Park, MD

More pre-publication
REVIEWS, COMMENTARIES, EVALUATIONS . . .

"Thoughtful and stimulating . . . tackles difficult issues. . . . Offers ideas, particularly in regard to preparing new professionals, that are practical and sometimes provocative, but clearly important for the continued growth of systems of care."

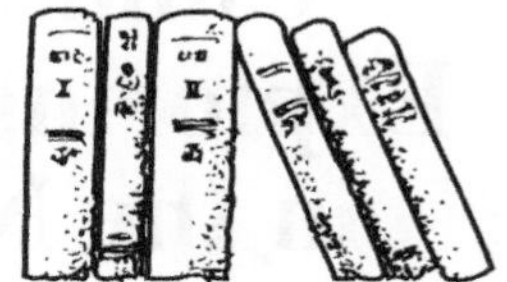

Robert M. Friedman, PhD
Professor and Chair
Department of Child and Family Studies
Louis de la Parte Florida Mental Health Institute,
University of South Florida

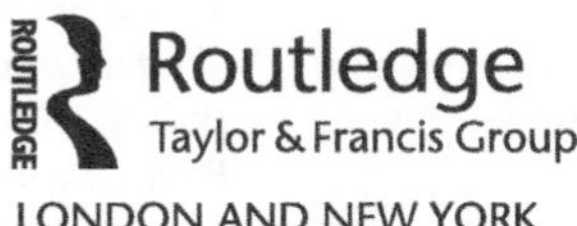

LONDON AND NEW YORK

Child Mental Health: Exploring Systems of Care in the New Millennium

Child Mental Health: Exploring Systems of Care in the New Millennium has been co-published simultaneously as *Journal of Family Social Work*, Volume 5, Number 3 2001.

The *Journal of Family Social Work* Monographic™ "Separates"

(formerly the *Journal of Social Work & Human Sexuality* series)*

For information on previous issues of the *Journal of Social Work & Human Sexuality* series, please contact: The Haworth Press, Inc., 10 Alice Street, Binghamton, NY 13904-1580 USA.

Below is a list of "separates," which in serials librarianship means a special issue simultaneously published as a special journal issue or double-issue *and* as a "separate" hardbound monograph. (This is a format which we also call a "DocuSerial.")

"Separates" are published because specialized libraries or professionals may wish to purchase a specific thematic issue by itself in a format which can be separately cataloged and shelved, as opposed to purchasing the journal on an on-going basis. Faculty members may also more easily consider a "separate" for classroom adoption.

"Separates" are carefully classified separately with the major book jobbers so that the journal tie-in can be noted on new book order slips to avoid duplicate purchasing.

You may wish to visit Haworth's website at . . .

http://www.HaworthPress.com

. . . to search our online catalog for complete tables of contents of these separates and related publications.

You may also call 1-800-HAWORTH (outside US/Canada: 607-722-5857), or Fax 1-800-895-0582 (outside US/Canada: 607-771-0012), or e-mail at:

getinfo@haworthpressinc.com

Child Mental Health: Exploring Systems of Care in the New Millennium, edited by David A. Dosser, Jr., PhD, Dorothea Handron, EdD, Susan McCammon, PhD, and John Y. Powell, PhD (Vol. 5, No. 3, 2001). *"Thoughtful and stimulating . . . tackles difficult issues . . . . Offers ideas, particularly in regard to preparing new professionals, that are practical and sometimes provocative, but clearly important for the continued growth of systems of care." (Robert M. Friedman, PhD, Professor and Chair, Department of Child and Family Studies, Louis de la Parte Florida Mental Health Institute, University of South Florida).*

Substance Abuse Issues Among Families in Diverse Populations, edited by Jorge Delva, PhD (Vol. 4, No. 4, 2000). *Discusses a variety of substance abuse issues including drug testing of welfare applicants as a requirement for benefits, parental substance abuse in African American and Latino families, and the perspectives of long-time Al-Anon members.*

Social Work and the Family Units, edited by David J. Ludwig, PhD, MDiv (Vol. 4, No. 3, 2000). *Offers therapists methods and suggestions for helping clients focus on problems within relationships and provides techniques and examples for conducting more successful and productive sessions.*

The Family, Spirituality, and Social Work, edited by Dorothy S. Becvar, MSW, PhD (Vol. 2, No. 4, 1998). *"This groundbreaking text is an evocative excursion into the realm of 'spirituality' within the domain of human services and treatment." (Marcia D. Brown-Standridge, ACSW, PhD, private practice, Terre Haute, Indiana)*

Cross-Cultural Practice with Couples and Families, edited by Philip M. Brown, PhD, LCSW, and John S. Shalett, MSW, BCSW (Vol. 2, No. 1/2, 1997). *"An excellent resource for practitioners and educators alike. It is an eye-opener and a first step in the process of understanding true diversity and cultural sensitivity." (Multicultural Review)*

Sexuality and Disabilities: A Guide for Human Service Practitioners, edited by Romel W. Mackelprang, DSW, MSW, and Deborah Valentine, PhD, MSW (Vol. 8, No. 2, 1993).* *"Emphasizes the need for individualized counseling in a supportive, educational context." (Science Books and Films)*

Adolescent Sexuality: New Challenges for Social Work, edited by Paula Allen-Meares, PhD, MSW, and Constance Hoenk Shapiro, PhD, MSW (Vol. 8, No. 1, 1989).* *"This is a valuable and wide-ranging* *look at the vital, complex, and very specific issues of adolescent sexuality and their implications for social work and social workers." (Paul H. Ephross, PhD, Professor, School of Social Work and Community Planning, University of Maryland at Baltimore)*

Treatment of Sex Offenders in Social Work and Mental Health Settings, edited by John S. Wodarski, PhD, and Daniel Whitaker, MSW (Vol. 7, No. 2, 1989).* *"The editors, besides contributing their own share of expertise, surrounded themselves with scientific experts who clearly enunciated their experiences in research design, data, conclusions, and applications." (Journal of the American Association of Psychiatric Administrators)*

The Sexually Unusual: Guide to Understanding and Helping, edited by Dennis M. Dailey, DSW (Vol. 7, No. 1, 1989).* *"If you want to know what you don't know about human sexual behavior, I challenge you to read this book, which is timely, cogent, and without a doubt, superior to any other book on this subject." (Arthur Herman, MSW, Chief Social Worker and Associate Director, Center for Sexual Health, Menninger Clinic, The Menninger Foundation, Topeka, Kansas)*

Sociological Aspects of Sexually Transmitted Diseases, edited by Margaret Rodway and Marianne Wright (Vol. 6, No. 2, 1988).* *"The most comprehensive resource guide on the topic of sexually transmitted diseases. It belongs in all the libraries of helping professionals and students, and is an up-to-date volume on an emerging issue in the field of human sexuality." (Professor Benjamin Schlesinger, Faculty of Social Work, University of Toronto, Canada; Author of Sexual Behavior in Canada (University of Toronto Press))*

Infertility and Adoption: A Guide for Social Work Practice, edited by Deborah Valentine (Vol. 6, No. 1, 1988).* *"Provides educators and practitioners with a rich compendium of information that will not only enhance their understanding of the dynamics involved in assessing and treating individuals and families presenting with concerns around fertility and adoption, but also provide an expanded context that takes into consideration program and policy issues." (Sadye L. Logan, DSW, Associate Professor, University of Kansas, School of Social Welfare)*

Intimate Relationships: Some Social Work Perspectives on Love, edited by Wendell Ricketts, BA, and Harvey Gochros, PhD (Vol. 5, No. 2, 1987).* *Insightful perspectives on the social worker's role in the counseling of clients who have problems with different kinds of love.*

Adolescent Sexualities: Overviews and Principles of Intervention, edited by Paula Allen-Meares, PhD, and David A. Shore, PhD (Vol. 5, No. 1, 1986).* *"The collection moves beyond many other articles and books by offering practical solutions and ideas for individuals working with adolescents." (SIECUS Report)*

Human Sexuality, Ethnoculture, and Social Work, edited by Larry Lister, DSW (Vol. 4, No. 3, 1987). **A valuable work providing basic cultural information within the context of human sexuality of several ethnocultural groups.*

Social Work Practice in Sexual Problems, edited by James Gripton, DSW, and Mary Valentich, PhD (Vol. 4, No. 1/2, 1986).* *"Serves as a valuable resource since it appears to encompass the major areas related to sexual problems." (Shankar A. Yelaja, DSW, Dean, Faculty of Social Work, Wilfrid Laurier University)*

Feminist Perspectives on Social Work and Human Sexuality, edited by Mary Valentich, PhD, and James Gripton, PhD, DSW (Vol. 3, No. 2/3, 1985).* *"Contains a powerful and unnerving message for educators, clinicians, and students. . . . important and useful . . . a valued addition to professional as well as academic libraries." (Canadian Social Work Review)*

Homosexuality and Social Work, edited by Robert Schoenberg, ACSW, and Richard S. Goldberg, MSS (Vol. 2, No. 2/3, 1984).* *"Packed with useful information on the special problems of both gay and lesbian clients. . . . A treasured resource for nurses, counselors, physicians, and other helping professionals." (Contemporary Sociology)*

Human Sexuality in Medical Social Work, edited by Larry Lister, DSW, and David A. Shore, PhD (Vol. 2, No. 1, 1984).* *"Excellently researched and written. . . . The role of the social worker as a member of the health care team is very well highlighted. . . . makes a valuable contribution to the counseling community." (Journal of Sex Education & Therapy)*

Social Work and Child Sexual Abuse, edited by Jon R. Conte, PhD, and David A. Shore, PhD (Vol. 1, No. 1/2, 1982).* *"This volume is a solid one, which contains a wealth of knowledge for the helping professional." (The Canadian Journal of Human Sexuality)*

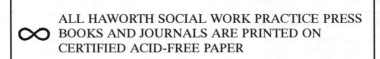

ALL HAWORTH SOCIAL WORK PRACTICE PRESS BOOKS AND JOURNALS ARE PRINTED ON CERTIFIED ACID-FREE PAPER

Child Mental Health: Exploring Systems of Care in the New Millennium

David A. Dosser, Jr., PhD
Dorothea Handron, EdD
Susan McCammon, PhD
John Y. Powell, PhD
Editors

Child Mental Health: Exploring Systems of Care in the New Millennium has been co-published simultaneously as *Journal of Family Social Work*, Volume 5, Number 3 2001.

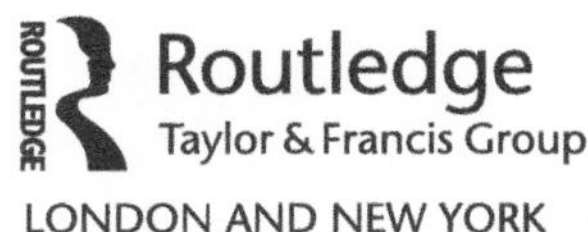

LONDON AND NEW YORK

Child Mental Health: Exploring Systems of Care in the New Millennium has been co-published simultaneously as *Journal of Family Social Work* ™, Volume 5, Number 3 2001.

First published 2001 by The Haworth Press

2 Park Square, Milton Park, Abingdon, Oxfordshire OX14 4RN
605 Third Avenue, New York, NY 10017

R*outledge is an imprint of the Taylor & Francis Group, an informa business*

First issued in hardback 2020

Copyright © 2001 Taylor & Francis

All rights reserved. No part of this book may be reprinted or reproduced or utilised in any form or by any electronic, mechanical, or other means, now known or hereafter invented, including photocopying and recording, or in any information storage or retrieval system, without permission in writing from the publishers.

Notice:
Product or corporate names may be trademarks or registered trademarks, and are used only for identification and explanation without intent to infringe.

Cover design by Thomas J. Mayshock Jr.

Library of Congress Cataloging-in-Publication Data

Child mental health : exploring systems of care in the new millennium / David A. Dosser, Jr. ... [et al.] editors.

p. cm.
"Co-published simultaneously as Journal of family social work, volume 5, number 3 2001."
Includes bibliographical references and index.
ISBN 0-7890-1380-0 (alk. paper)–ISBN 0-7890-1381-9 (pbk. : alk. paper)
1. Child mental health. 2. Child mental health services I. Dosser, Daivd A.

RJ499 .C4846 2001
362.2′083–dc21 2001024983

ISBN: 978-0-7890-1380-4 (hbk)

Indexing, Abstracting & Website/Internet Coverage

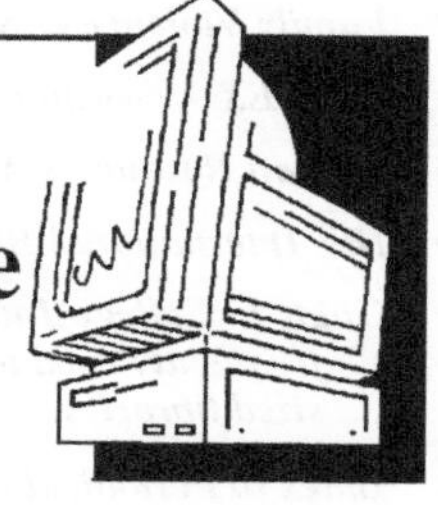

This section provides you with a list of major indexing & abstracting services. That is to say, each service began covering this periodical during the year noted in the right column. Most Websites which are listed below have indicated that they will either post, disseminate, compile, archive, cite or alert their own Website users with research-based content from this work. (This list is as current as the copyright date of this publication.)

Abstracting, Website/Indexing Coverage	Year When Coverage Began
• *Abstracts in Anthropology*	**1995**
• *Abstracts in Social Gerontology: Current Literature on Aging*	**1995**
• *AgeLine Database*	**1999**
• *Applied Social Sciences Index & Abstracts (ASSIA) (Online: ASSI via Data-Star) (CDRom: ASSIA Plus) <http://www.bowker-saur.co.uk>*	**1995**
• *BUBL Information Service: An Internet-based Information Service for the UK higher education community <URL: http://bubl.ac.uk/>*	**1996**
• *Cambridge Scientific Abstracts <www.csa.com>*	**1995**
• *caredata CD: the social & community care database*	**1995**
• *CINAHL (Cumulative Index to Nursing & Allied Health Literature), in print, EBSCO, and SilverPlatter, Data-Star, and PaperChase. (Support materials include Subject Heading List, Database Search Guide, and instructional video)*	**1995**
• *CNPIEC Reference Guide: Chinese National Directory of Foreign Periodicals*	**1996**
• *Criminal Justice Abstracts*	**1995**
• *Educational Administration Abstracts (EAA)*	**1995**
• *Family Studies Database (online and CD/ROM) <www.nisc.com>*	**1996**

(continued)

- *Family Violence & Sexual Assault Bulletin* **1995**
- *FINDEX <www.publist.com>* **1999**
- *Human Resources Abstracts (HRA)* **1995**
- *IBZ International Bibliography of Periodical Literature* **1994**
- *Guide to College Journals (core list compiled by integrating 48 indexes frequently used to support undergraduate programs in small to medium sized libraries* **1999**
- *Index to Periodical Articles Related to Law* **1995**
- *National Criminal Justice Reference Service* **1999**
- *Periodica Islamica* **1994**
- *Psychological Abstracts (PsycINFO)* **1995**
- *Referativnyi Zhurnal (Abstracts Journal of the All-Russian Institute of Scientific and Technical Information-in Russian)* **1994**
- *Sage Family Studies Abstracts (SFSA)* **1995**
- *Social Services Abstracts <www.csa.com>* **1995**
- *Social Work Abstracts* **1995**
- *Sociological Abstracts (SA) <www.csa.com>* **1995**
- *Studies on Women Abstracts* **1995**
- *Violence and Abuse Abstracts: A Review of Current Literature on Interpersonal Violence (VAA)* **1995**

Special Bibliographic Notes related to special journal issues (separates) and indexing/abstracting:

- indexing/abstracting services in this list will also cover material in any "separate" that is co-published simultaneously with Haworth's special thematic journal issue or DocuSerial. Indexing/abstracting usually covers material at the article/chapter level.
- monographic co-editions are intended for either non-subscribers or libraries which intend to purchase a second copy for their circulating collections.
- monographic co-editions are reported to all jobbers/wholesalers/approval plans. The source journal is listed as the "series" to assist the prevention of duplicate purchasing in the same manner utilized for books-in-series.
- to facilitate user/access services all indexing/abstracting services are encouraged to utilize the co-indexing entry note indicated at the bottom of the first page of each article/chapter/contribution.
- this is intended to assist a library user of any reference tool (whether print, electronic, online, or CD-ROM) to locate the monographic version if the library has purchased this version but not a subscription to the source journal.
- individual articles/chapters in any Haworth publication are also available through the Haworth Document Delivery Service (HDDS).

Child Mental Health: Exploring Systems of Care in the New Millennium

CONTENTS

ABOUT THE EDITORS

David A. Dosser, Jr., PhD, is Associate Professor and Director of the Marriage and Family Therapy Program in the School of Human Environmental Sciences at East Carolina University. Dr. Dosser is a clinical member and approved supervisor in the American Association for Marriage and Family Therapy and Chair of the North Carolina Marriage and Family Therapy Licensure Board. His recent publications include *Challenges of Interdisciplinary Collaboration: A Faculty Consortium's Initial Attempts to Model Collaborative Practice; Wraparound–The Wave of the Future: Theoretical and Professional Practice Implications for Children and Families with Complex Needs*; and *Toward the Development of Ethical Guidelines for Family Preservation.* Dr. Dosser is a licensed marriage and family therapist. He maintains an active practice in systemic therapy with couples and families at East Carolina University's Family Therapy Clinic.

Dorothea Handron, EdD, is Associate Professor in the Department of Community and Mental Health Nursing and Nursing Services Administration. She is certified by the ANCC as a clinical specialist in adult psychiatric/mental health nursing. Dr. Handron teaches graduate courses in advanced practice in psychiatric nursing, child/family mental health services, interdisciplinary education, and family theory. Her work has appeared in the professional journals *Perspectives in Psychiatric Care, The Diabetes Educator, The Nurse Practitioner*, and *The American Journal of Primary Health Care.*

Susan McCammon, PhD, is Professor of Psychology and Director of the Eastern North Carolina Public Academic Liaison, which promotes curriculum development and training for improving the system of care for children with serious emotional problems and their families. She teaches in the MA program in clinical psychology and consults with child and family services at the local community mental health center. She currently teaches courses in child and family therapeutic interventions, interdisciplinary practice, and sexual behavior. Her research interests include children's mental health, coping with trauma, human sexuality, and women's studies. She is co-author of the textbook, *Making Choices in Sexuality: Research and Applications.*

John Y. Powell, PhD, is Professor, Child and Family Area of Specialization, in the Master of Social Work Program at East Carolina University. He is licensed both as a clinical social worker and as a marriage and family therapist. Dr. Powell is the author of *Family-Centered Practice in Residential Treatment* (The Haworth Press, Inc.). In 1999, he received the "Champion of the Family Award" from the North Carolina Association for Marriage and Family Therapy.

Foreword: Preparing Practitioners for an Evolving System of Care

During the past decade, our care of children with serious emotional challenges has undergone a dramatic shift in both theory and practice. What has evolved is a system of care that encompasses a coordinated spectrum of services and supports that are responsive to the dynamic needs of children and families. Values and principles for the system of care have been clearly articulated and serve to guide our work to be child-centered and family-focused, community-based, and culturally sensitive. A primary voice in helping to shape this system of care has been the families, the consumers of mental health services and treatment.

The foundation on which the system of care is built involves families and practitioners *partnering* at all levels throughout the system, from policy development to service and treatment planning to program evaluation. Instead of viewing families as recipients of mental health services that practitioners control, the paradigm has shifted to including families as key participants and decision-makers. This paradigm shift has been a sometimes grueling learning process for both practitioners and families, given our training and long-standing approach to care. The articles in this volume are a collection of papers primarily based out of work at East Carolina University in Greenville, North Carolina that examine elements of the system of care in relation to the training needs of practitioners to prepare them to work effectively within a collaborative and interdisciplinary system.

McGinty, McCammon, and Koeppen have provided readers with an excellent working model of a wraparound process, the hallmark of the system of care. Through their description and assessment of the process, they identify several barriers to effective wraparound that are based in practitioners' lack

---

[Haworth co-indexing entry note]: "Foreword: Preparing Practitioners for an Evolving System of Care." De Carolis, Gary. Co-published simultaneously in *Journal of Family Social Work* (The Haworth Social Work Practice Press, an imprint of The Haworth Press, Inc.) Vol. 5, No. 3, 2001, pp. xiii-xv; and: *Child Mental Health: Exploring Systems of Care in the New Millennium* (ed: David A. Dosser, Jr. et al.) The Haworth Social Work Practice Press, an imprint of The Haworth Press, Inc., 2001, pp. xiii-xv. Single or multiple copies of this article are available for a fee from The Haworth Document Delivery Service [1-800-342-9678, 9:00 a.m. - 5:00 p.m. (EST). E-mail address: getinfo@haworthpressinc.com].

of training in family-centered and strength-based processes which also effect policy and funding structures. In a similar vein, McCammon, Spencer, and Friesen discuss the need to help social workers learn parent partnering skills and the potential roles that families can play in the system of care. An additional area in which practitioners lack training and experience is addressed by Dosser, Smith, Markowski, and Cain. They suggest that little training is provided in assessing, understanding, and integrating a family's spiritual beliefs as natural supports that are culturally and ecologically oriented.

It is evident that parent-practitioner partnerships require special skills to reach a depth that results in effective relationships and positive outcomes. In addition, because the system of care seeks to coordinate and integrate services and treatment, practitioners must also develop relationships and collaborations with each other. Powell, Privette, Miller, and Whittaker point out that practitioners are typically trained in specific models related to their discipline, and not trained in team approaches to service delivery. As a result, effective collaboration is sometimes prevented because of lack of understanding of or experience with other disciplines.

As aptly stated by McCammon et al. in reference to family member roles and the system of care, " . . . this movement has outstripped professional training and practice." Fortunately, our training institutions are beginning to examine their programs in relation to the characteristics of the system of care so that practitioners will emerge with skills that prepare them to effectively engage with families and other providers. Handron and Diamond suggest that there are many challenges to changing mental health education that will require an invested faculty with time to build relationships. Faculty will face such barriers as competitive behaviors, the complexity of scheduling courses across disciplines, the expense of multiple teachers for single courses, curriculum biases, and the basic need to relinquish any supremacy of theory.

In their article on an "Interdisciplinary Helping Process Framework," Powell et al. describe how they developed an interdisciplinary, collaborative practice course at East Carolina University that is taught by a team of faculty from a cross-section of disciplines. Key to the development of the curriculum was the need to first establish a *unifying* framework for collaborative, interdisciplinary practice and professional-consumer partnerships. By sponsoring an academic symposium, the University brought together speakers who had written and spoken about therapeutic models that are based upon relationship building and social ecology. These theories interface with the system of care values and principles, providing a helpful framework for practitioners. They emphasize the importance of consumers driving the change process and giving feedback about their expectations, the process, and outcomes.

Families have many potential roles in the system of care, which have been eloquently described by McCammon et al. in their article on "Promoting Family Empowerment." Like East Carolina University, other training institutions will be well served to include families as integral educators and trainers of practitioners at the pre-service and graduate levels. The authors suggest that because family members provoke positive change in policies, they can be significant contributors to change in training curricula.

Pierpont, Pozzuto, and Powell designed a service learning assignment for their social work students to help them understand social policy and its impact on consumers, linking it to advocacy and practice. This unique type of experiential training provides opportunities for students to learn from consumers and recognizes their value in changing harmful policies and programs. Another important training strategy suggested by Handron et al. is to provide shared classroom experiences for cross-discipline students early in training programs so that the team approach to service delivery is explored and integrated into future thinking.

Finally, Bass, Dosser, and Powell propose teaching a schema as a tool that will support both practitioners and consumers in shifting their thinking from a provider-as-expert role to one of building partnerships. Recognizing the importance of language in communicating beliefs and expectations, the authors identify six steps that are characterized by the key words "joining," "discovery," "changing," "celebrating," "separating," and "reflection." As our training institutions move towards changing their curricula and teaching strategies to meet the needs of the system of care, these words should guide them in their own efforts.

We celebrate the authors who have contributed to this volume in their efforts to support change, and thank them for their desire to improve the care we provide to our children and their families.

Gary De Carolis, Chief
Child, Adolescent and Family Branch
Federal Center for Mental Health Services
Substance Abuse & Mental Health Services Administration
Rockville, MD

Promoting Family Empowerment Through Multiple Roles

Susan L. McCammon, PhD
Sandra A. Spencer, BA
Barbara J. Friesen, PhD

SUMMARY. A guiding principle in the system of care philosophy for meeting the needs of children with serious emotional problems and their families is that the families "should be full participants in all aspects of the planning and delivery of services" (Stroul & Friedman, 1996, p. 9). Family members, both individually and as representatives of family organizations, are participating in systems of care in a number

---

Susan L. McCammon is Professor, Department of Psychology, East Carolina University and Director, the Social Sciences Training Consortium. Sandra A. Spencer is Executive Director, WE CARE, Greenville, NC. Barbara J. Friesen is Professor, School of Social Work, Portland State University, and Center Director, Research and Training Center, Regional Research Institute for Human Services.

Address correspondence to: Susan L. McCammon, Department of Psychology, Rawl Building, East Carolina University, Greenville, NC 27858-4353 (E-mail: mccammons@mail.ecu.edu).

Preparation of this manuscript was supported in part by a contract between the North Carolina Division of MH/DD/SAS, Child and Family Services Section and the East Carolina University Social Sciences Training Consortium. Support for manuscript preparation was also provided by Ms. Traci Lynch. Support was also provided from funding from the National Institute on Disability and Rehabilitation Research, United States Department of Education, and the Center for Mental Health Services, Substance Abuse Mental Health Services Administration, United States Department of Health and Human Services (Grant #H133B990025). The contents of this publication do not necessarily reflect the views or policies of the funding agencies.

[Haworth co-indexing entry note]: "Promoting Family Empowerment Through Multiple Roles." McCammon, Susan L., Sandra A. Spencer, and Barbara J. Friesen. Co-published simultaneously in *Journal of Family Social Work* (The Haworth Social Work Practice Press, an imprint of The Haworth Press, Inc.) Vol. 5, No. 3, 2001, pp. 1-24; and: *Child Mental Health: Exploring Systems of Care in the New Millennium* (ed: David A. Dosser, Jr. et al.) The Haworth Social Work Practice Press, an imprint of The Haworth Press, Inc., 2001, pp. 1-24. Single or multiple copies of this article are available for a fee from The Haworth Document Delivery Service [1-800-342-9678, 9:00 a.m. - 5:00 p.m. (EST). E-mail address: getinfo@haworthpressinc.com].

© 2001 by The Haworth Press, Inc. All rights reserved.

of vital roles. Friesen and Stephens (1998) delineated six of these roles, and summarized related practice and research. In this paper we expand and continue their discussion of multiple roles, adding a seventh with elaboration of the role of family members as educators and trainers, separating that from the role of service provider. The following roles are reviewed: family members as context; targets for change and recipients of service; partners in the treatment process; service providers; educators and trainers of professionals, students, and other family members; advocates and policymakers; and evaluators and researchers. Recognition of these expanded family roles may help service providers be better prepared to work collaboratively with families and family organizations, and to become aware of the accomplishments that may be achieved through such collaboration. *[Article copies available for a fee from The Haworth Document Delivery Service: 1-800-342-9678. E-mail address: <getinfo@haworthpressinc.com> Website: <http://www.HaworthPress.com> © 2001 by The Haworth Press, Inc. All rights reserved.]*

KEYWORDS. Family empowerment, parent-professional collaboration

One of the guiding principles of a system of care for meeting the needs of children with serious emotional problems and their families is that the families "should be full participants in all aspects of the planning and delivery of services" (Stroul & Friedman, 1996, p. 9). (In using the term "families" we refer not only to biological nuclear families, but also extended kin caregivers as well as foster and adoptive families.) Increasingly, families are being seen as their children's most important resource, and even the most troubled are viewed as having strengths to be built upon (Stroul, Friedman, Hernandez, Roebuck, Lourie & Koyanagi, 1996). In fact, DeChillo, Koren and Schultze (1994) suggested that the degree to which various helping professions are able to promote true collaboration with families will largely determine how much progress can be accomplished in meeting the needs of such children and their families.

The "competence paradigm" advocated by Marsh (1996) assumes that families are basically competent in their functioning, and that the role of professionals should be to assist the families in meeting their own goals and to empower them to achieve mastery and control over their life circumstances. However, traditional training programs have been very limited in their efforts to prepare professionals to collaborate with family members and pool efforts with them to improve the system of care in children's mental health (Jivanjee & Friesen, 1997). A parent-professional partnership model has been called for, in which parents surpass the traditional role of "patients" or "clients" to assume a partnership or collaborative role. The last decade has hosted an evolution in the way families are viewed in systems of care. Families have been involved in the development, implementation, and evaluation of such systems. Systems of care promote family participation, and families are empowered. Families play out this empowerment as they develop advocacy skills, a sense of self-efficacy, and the ability to access needed services and supports.

As family members are better able to care for their children, they become increasingly more involved in building these systems of care to help other families. Professionals are now recognizing the experience they bring to the table as valuable. These professionals are beginning to seek out the expertise of family members. A need for support to families rearing children with serious emotional and mental health challenges has sparked a national family movement. Family-run organizations have emerged throughout the country, resulting in a strong family voice. "As families have come together for mutual support and sharing information, many have 'gone public' with their perspectives on the current system and their demands for better services" (Friesen & Wahlers, 1993).

While the roles of family members within state-level and local systems of care have expanded, as Friesen and Stephens (1998) noted, this movement has outstripped professional training and practice. They outlined six broad role sets in which family members are involved, and summarized research and practice examples. Given this dramatic role expansion, the training of social workers and other service providers needs to include information that will better prepare them to work collaboratively with families and family organizations.

In this article, we continue the Friesen and Stephens (1998) description of multiple roles, update the research summary, and draw further practice and training implications for professionals for realizing their possibilities and responsibilities in implementing this partnership model. We provide examples of programs which offer support and consultation to promote family participation in multiple roles. In addition, we highlight the expertise and contributions to systems of care which can be tapped by family participation across these roles.

The roles to be examined include the six identified by Friesen and Stephens (1998), and adding a seventh with elaboration of the role of family member as educator and trainer, separating that from service provider. The roles include the following: family members as context; targets for change and recipients of service; partners in the treatment process; service providers, including consultants; educators and trainers of professionals, students, and other family members; advocates and policymakers; and evaluators and researchers.

FAMILY MEMBERS AS CONTEXT

The initial family role identified by Friesen and Stephens (1998) was that of family members as context, in which family members are viewed as a crucial component of the environment of a child who has emotional or behavioral problems. Much of the past focus on this role has identified parents, through "ineffective or malevolent parenting," as likely causal agents in their children's mental health problems (Friesen & Stephens, 1998, p. 232). Psychoanalytic theories addressing early childhood development, and family systems theories interpreting some mental illnesses as an " 'adaptation' to dysfunction in the parents," often stigmatized parents and offered little practical assistance (Riesser & Schorske, 1994). Current environmental approaches, based on a diathesis-stress model, acknowledge biological vulnerabilities to stress in people with mental health problems, and focus on ways to alter the environment to reduce and manage crises (Riesser & Schorske, 1994).

Contemporary conceptualizations of the family environment of persons with persistent emotional problems or mental illness have begun focusing on the concept of "family burden." This literature has grown in the wake of deinstitutionalization, with recognition of the need for families to attempt to fill the gaps between the promise and the reality of care for mentally ill family members (Riesser & Schorske, 1994). " 'Family burden' has come to describe an extensive literature on the felt experience of families in coping with the acute and long-term responsibilities associated with an inadequate system of community care and treatment" (p. 10). The burdens include disruptions to daily family life, worry and a sense of loss, social isolation, and financial expense. While earlier studies of family burden focused on caregivers of mentally ill adults, the elderly, or children with chronic physical illness, recent studies have investigated the experiences of parents of children with psychiatric, emotional, and behavioral problems.

These studies have addressed "parental burden" (Angold, Messer, Stangl, Farmer, Costello, & Burns, 1998), also referred to as "caregiver strain" (Brannan, Heflinger, & Bickman, 1997)) or more broadly, "family impact" (Farmer, Burns, Angold & Costello, 1997). While adults caring for children with an emotional disability have reported more frequent stressors than parents from a general population sample, many would bristle at the characterization of their child as a "burden." In fact, many have reported ways in which caring for their child with special needs has enriched their lives (Yatchmenoff, Koren, Friesen, Gordon, & Kinney, 1998).

In the Great Smoky Mountains Study, a longitudinal study of 4500 families in western North Carolina, parents were asked to identify perceived burdens resulting from their children's psychiatric symptoms. Parents whose children had a diagnosis and impairment were most likely to report burdens (38.8%), including effects on personal well-being, stigma, and restrictions on personal activities (Angold et al., 1998). However, parent perception of burden was the most important predictor of seeking specialty mental health service (above the amount and type of symptoms). If parents felt burden from their child's symptoms, they were much more likely to seek services for them.

The Fort Bragg Evaluation Project assessed families participating in the Civilian Health and Medical Program of the Uniformed Services mental health benefits for dependent children program. In three CHAMPUS-defined catchment areas which were studied, families were especially likely to report subjective, as opposed to objective, strain. This included such items as worry about their child and family's future, feeling sad or unhappy, and tired or strained (Brannan et al., 1997), as well as feeling negatively toward the child or his/her behavior.

Similarly, Yatchmenoff et al. (1998) found stress across many aspects of respondents' lives in their study of the experiences of 214 families in which there was a child with a serious emotional disorder. Families felt the greatest degree of stress when their child's disorder was more severe, caregivers felt less empowered, and there was a lack of coordination among service providers. They did, however, also find that some families reported enrichment from their caregiving experience. Enrichment was related to feeling empowered ("a sense of competence and confidence in their ability to deal with problems"), and having spiritual support.

Across these studies, families whose children had the greatest functional impairments and the highest problem or symptom scores reported greater caregiver strain. Furthermore, elevated caregiver strain was associated with use of inpatient hospitalization and extended use of intermediate services such as in-home and day treatment services (Brannan et al., 1997). Given the centrality of family caregivers in bringing children to treatment, making and following through on treatment plans, and in supporting gains in the natural environment, caregiver strain has important implications for clinical outcomes (Brannan et al., 1997).

Although those who have done burden research have called for professionals working in hospitals and community clinics to provide burden alleviation services, this has not become common practice (Johnson, 1994). The burden amelioration interventions reported in the adult literature focus mainly on psychoeducational interventions with families and extensive case management. These have been shown to reduce relapses. In the child services literature, rather than conceptualized as "burden amelioration," interventions with similar goals are directed toward providing "family support." For example, in three Oregon counties, paraprofessionals served as Family Associates, serving families by offering information, emotional support and help with service barriers such as transportation and childcare for siblings (Koroloff, Elliott, Koren & Friesen, 1996). The intervention had a moderate effect, in comparison to service use patterns in four other counties. The intervention families were more likely to make and keep an initial appointment at the mental health clinic, and to report higher rates of empowerment (sense of mastery and ability to cope with difficult situations) at post-test.

The Finger Lakes Family Support Project is an example of a professional family-support program (Friesen & Wahlers, 1993). This program is based on the concept of providing "whatever it takes" to meet the social, emotional, and tangible needs of families. Project evaluation documented a decrease over time in parenting stress and parent ratings of the severity of their child's problem severity. Researchers concluded that "family-support services can help change the lives of family members from feeling over-stressed and desperate to empowered and hopeful" (p. 15).

The type of family empowerment in the "family as context" literature focuses mainly on the personal level of empowerment, as described by Heflinger and Bickman (1996). At this level, promoting family empowerment focuses on increasing knowledge (about the mental health system, diagnoses, parental rights, etc.), skills (communication, problem-solving, resource identification), and self-efficacy (feeling capable). While these outcomes are critical and necessary, Heflinger and Bickman noted their insufficiency. Merely enhancing a sense of personal control, when there is no actual control, typically supports the status quo or promotes conflict. Therefore, empowerment strategies must also promote a process that increases access to resources; enhances ability to influence people, organizations, and policies; and "aspires toward more cooperative and collaborative parent-professional interaction" (p. 105).

FAMILY MEMBERS AS TARGETS FOR CHANGE AND SERVICE RECIPIENTS

The role of "target for change" or service recipient probably constitutes the main way in which family members are involved in their children's treatment (Friesen & Stephens, 1998). Marsh (1994) recommended that a full continuum of family-oriented services, including nonclinical services (education and support) and clinical services (therapy and psychoeducation) be available for serving families of people with serious mental illness. A comprehensive program of nonclinical services should include the following: (a) didactic information about serious emotional disturbance and the mental health system; (b) skills training in communication, resolution of conflict, problem solving, assertiveness, behavior management, and stress management; (c) opportunity for processing and sharing such emotions; (d) a focus on the family process of coping with mental illness and its impact on the family; and (e) a focus on increasing the use of informal and formal support networks.

Parent training is often recommended to improve caregivers' basic parenting skills or to teach specific behavior management techniques (Friesen & Stephens, 1998), but is frequently perceived by consumers to be offered from a "pathology" perspective. However, some parents do need help with the basic skills of daily living, effective parenting, and promoting their child's development. An example of a multi-program family center that offers help with these tasks in the context of nurturing, supportive relationships is Peanut Butter and Jelly (PB & J), in Albuquerque, New Mexico (Ruiz et al., 1997). By offering parenting skills training, and activities to strengthen parent-child communication and bonding, in the context of a culturally sensitive center that focuses holistically on the needs of families, PB & J programs come across as empowering and supportive to families.

Another type of family education and training strategy, that of reducing "expressed emotion" (EE) (expression of highly critical, hostile, or emotionally over-involved attitudes) towards a mentally ill family member, was based on the idea that families in high EE homes are more stressful than supportive for schizophrenic or manic persons, and promote relapse. However, recent discussion of the family EE concept suggested that EE may reflect a more reciprocal process of influence between the identified patient and the family, and that it is amenable to educational intervention about mental illness (McFarlane & Lukens, 1994). McFarlane and Lukens recommended intervention at several systemic levels: medication and social skills training to reduce symptoms and problem behaviors; family psychoeducation to give accurate information and correct misattribution regarding behaviors; multiple family groups to reduce isolation and stigma, and share coping strategies; and community education to decrease stigma and increase rehabilitation opportunities. They suggested that we are now in an era in which the complexity of the family with a mentally ill person is recognized, and that there is now more focus on designing acceptable and effective strategies for providing assistance.

FAMILY MEMBERS AS PARTNERS IN THE TREATMENT PROCESS

In this role parents and other caregivers have active involvement in planning, implementing, and evaluating services for their child with an emotional disorder, as well as for the rest of the family. For caregivers, such participation involves working collaboratively with service providers to identify mutual goals, plan services based on the child and family's needs, strengths, and preferences, observe and report about how the plan is working, and support the youth's participation in the program developed for him/her.

For service providers, working collaboratively with families often represents a shift from traditional direct practice roles to acting as facilitators, guides, and coaches. These ideas are entirely compatible with social work values and practice approaches such as "competency-based" (Moore-Kirkland, 1981), "strengths-based" (Saleeby, 1996), and "empowerment" (Dunlap, 1997; Lee, 1994; Pinderhughes, 1995). Indeed, social workers and other practitioners in the area of children's mental health sometimes ask, "what's new?" asserting that their practice already reflects the values and principles of collaborative practice.

Contrary to these practitioners' beliefs, however, studies examining family members' perspectives reveal that collaboration is still more of a goal than a reality in many settings (Cournoyer & Johnson, 1991; DeChillo et al., 1994; Friesen, Koren, & Koroloff, 1992; Simpson, Koroloff, Friesen, & Gac, 1999). This discrepancy between practitioners' and family members' views may have a number of explanations. The possibilities include: (1) some service providers still work within very traditional "expert-client" practice frameworks; (2) some practitioners do, indeed, engage in collaborative practices, but not with sufficient depth or consistency to meet family members' expectations; (3) the intentions of professionals are collaborative, but practices associated with their theoretical frameworks lead them to behave in ways that family members don't perceive as collaborative (Johnson, Cournoyer, & Fisher, 1994); and/or (4) because of previous negative experiences, family members may misinterpret neutral or ambiguous behavior on the part of practitioners as blaming or condescending.

Several related practitioner attitudes and behaviors appear to be key to collaborative practice. The first is *sensitivity to the stigma and blame* felt by many families of children with emotional, behavioral, or mental disorders. Manifestations of this sensitivity include the avoidance of interactions that may be interpreted or misunderstood as blaming, such as taking in-depth social and psychological histories during initial interviews, which many families experience as confirmation of their fears that "it's all my fault" (Friesen & Huff, 1996).

A second important area is *genuine mutuality in identifying needs, setting goals, and planning and developing services*. This entails working with families and youth to define their needs as they see them, and locating or developing appropriate services. This family-centered, "whatever it takes" approach calls for considerable practice flexibility, and is characteristic of wraparound services (Burchard & Clarke, 1990; Burns & Goldman, 1999; VanDenBerg & Grealish, 1996) that have gained much currency in the children's mental health field over the last 15 years. This framework can be contrasted with "program-centered services" that seek a match between client needs and existing services, but may lack the capacity to respond to the unique needs of children and families (Friesen & Huff, 1996).

An illustration of this point is reported by Thomas and Friesen (1990). In this example, a single, working mother of three approached a mental health clinic for help getting her 7-year-old child ready for school in the mornings. Her son had extreme difficulty sustaining attention, and his inability to get ready without constant supervision was having a negative effect on the entire family. His mother felt that without assistance she could not cope with this problem and keep her job. The intake social worker at the mental health clinic explained that they did not have such a service, but offered counseling since the mother was so distraught. The social worker in this case was not engaged in "bad practice," in fact, she was trying to be helpful by offering what was available. From the family member's perspective, however, the service that was offered not only did not meet her need, but shifted the focus from her request for a needed service to her own psychological functioning. The mother agreed that she was feeling extremely frustrated with her son, and with the effect that his behavior was having on the entire family, but her belief was that her desperation would be reduced by help getting her son ready for school. The parent felt blamed, that she had not been listened to or heard, that her needs had not been addressed, and she could see no reason to return to the mental health clinic. Supportive counseling might also have been helpful, but the mother was not receptive to such suggestions until her immediate need was addressed. This example illustrates the gap that often occurs between parents' needs and goals, and the response of the service system.

A third related area is the *centrality of the family in decision-making* in all aspects of the treatment process, honoring the family's definition of the problem and choices about the type, location, frequency, and duration of services. Acting on this principle may require that practitioners reorient their ideas about power and professional authority. This topic sometimes elicits concern on the part of practitioners that power sharing may involve inappropriate abdication of professional authority. This concern, we believe, flows from a "fixed pie" view of power (Erchul & Raven, 1997; Hasenfeld, 1987) that is not the experience of practitioners and family members who have successfully learned to function as partners (Williams-Murphy, DeChillo, Koren, & Hunter, 1994). Helping parents retain or regain their parental authority through respecting and supporting their right to make crucial decisions regarding their children and families does not diminish the need for professional expertise, and may actually enhance understanding between families and practitioners. As Moore-Kirkland (1981) pointed out, what may be labeled as resistance on the part of families may in fact be a discrepancy between the goals of the family and the goals of the practitioner. Tannen

(1996) made a similar point, suggesting that "resistant" families may, in fact, be appropriately cautious, and that their objections are a signal that mutual goal-setting did not occur.

The concept of partnership has proven more difficult to implement than to describe. Simpson et al. (1999) interviewed family members and service providers from more than 20 community-based systems of care for children and families. They identified as a major challenge, "a lack of agreement among family members and providers on how collaboration is defined and practiced . . . and more particularly, agreement on how power is shared" (p. 109). Some families and practitioners have a vision of a "50/50" partnership, with decisions and responsibilities shared equally across time, while others envision something more like a "limited" partnership, where one partner (either the family or the professional) has the controlling interest. In reality, a dynamic distribution of responsibility changing, according to the needs, resources, and circumstances of the family, characterizes successful partnerships.

The role of family members in program- or system-level evaluation is discussed in a subsequent section of this article. It is important to note here, however, that the responsiveness of practitioners to feedback from family members and youth about how well plans are working was found by DeChillo et al. (1994) to be one of the factors that distinguished family members' descriptions of collaborative practice from those of the least collaborative professional with whom they had worked.

FAMILY MEMBERS AS SERVICE PROVIDERS

Family members of children with emotional and behavioral challenges have long been providing services to their own and other families through self-help (providing emotional support, self-education, and advice), as well as performing service coordination functions (Ignelzi & Dague, 1995). The next step in the evolution of parent involvement has been parents providing these and other direct services for pay. Ignelzi and Dague identified a number of roles in which parents have served as paid providers: mentors, case managers, early intervention workers, advocates, in-home support staff, respite providers, service planners, and managers of family cash grants. Recently described examples of family-professional collaboration show the continuing development of parents in service-provision roles.

Initiatives in Illinois and Rhode Island are using parents as system of care facilitators (Osher et al., 1999). The role of Parent Resource Developer evolved through several titles and job descriptions in the Community Wraparound Initiative in LaGrange, Illinois. These providers are employed through the Illinois Federation of Families for Children's Mental Health, and are co-supervised by the Federation as well as the clinical director of the agency in which they work. Families being served through the initiative reported that following six months of working with a Family Resource Developer they increased their knowledge regarding their children's disabilities and how to care for them and obtain services. They were also helped to obtain needed financial assistance from public agencies and home-based services. REACH Rhode Island employs Family Service Coordinators, who are seen as the most essential feature of the project and the source of its success.

The Philadelphia Youth Advocate Program summer day camp offers a program that is designed and partially staffed by family members (Osher et al., 1998). This camp is funded through a local Medicaid behavioral managed-care organization, and is in its seventh year. It includes an arts focus to fit the needs and backgrounds of children in the South Philadelphia community by helping children compose, conduct, and perform their own musical and dramatic productions.

Parent Connections in Baltimore, Maryland offers another example of parents as providers. Their trained Parent Mentors receive an hourly stipend for working up to ten hours a week. The Mentors are parents or long-term guardians of adult children who received treatment between the ages of nine and fourteen for a mental, emotional, or behavioral disorder. The impact of the program is being studied in a randomized trial in which participating families, in addition to whatever formal mental health services they receive, are assigned to either Parent Connections (experimental group) or a Parent Resource Awareness Program (control group) (Sakwa & Ireys, 1998). The investigators anticipate that the special support and guidance of the peer mentors will facilitate enhanced mental health outcomes for both children and parents.

FAMILY MEMBERS AS EDUCATORS AND CONSULTANTS

As many as six million children in the United States may have a serious emotional disturbance (Center for Mental Health Services, 1996), and are in need of treatment. Educating the public and removing stigma around children's mental health is very important to families raising children with serious emotional, behavioral, and mental health issues. Training on these issues has become one of the main missions of family-run organizations. In many cases, the training started in families gathering at family support group meetings and telling their stories. Families started to support each other, telling of success in accessing services or in improving the life of their child. Family organizations turned this support into training curricula. The unique experience and perspective that family members had in accessing services, and rearing children with complex mental health needs, provided a basis for training curricula which became a valuable tool in training both family members and providers. Family members were able to tell providers what they perceived as barriers to using those agencies' services. Family members and family-run organizations serve as trainers, educators and consultants to the same systems that were treating their child and family.

There is little research on the impact of family members' training providers. In 1987, the Research and Training Center on Family Support initiated a curriculum and training program on parent-professional partnership. The curriculum, "Working Together," consisted of training teams of one parent and one professional. What this project revealed was that collaboration sounded fine in theory, but was very hard to implement (Koroloff, Friesen, Reilly, & Rinkin, 1996).

Hawaii Families as Allies, a family-run organization in Hawaii, started this same way; they offered support to families. Families in need of support attended meetings with other family members who had been using the system for a while. This support turned into training. Hawaii Families as Allies developed two curricula, "Developing Families as Allies" and "Impact on Families." This family-run organization was able to receive funding and later involved providers in the training. Today, Hawaii Families as Allies has a total of 16 curricula they offer statewide.

Parents have also been active as educators on university campuses (Osher, deFur, Nava, Spencer, & Toth-Dennis, 1999). In Maine, Parent Advocate Specialists, and family members from the community of Washington County, guest lecture in university classes. At the University of Maine at Machais, family members share their stories in an educational psychology class that is a required course for all education majors. At the University of Maine at Orono family members are sharing their experience in the School of Social Work. Parents of children with emotional and behavioral disabilities teach a two-hour class session to social work graduate students at the University of Connecticut. In addition, the instructors require a written assignment in which students integrate what they learned in the class session with assigned readings from the parent-professional collaboration literature. Johnson (2000) examined the impact of this module across nine classes and found that parent blaming attitudes decreased. She also found that students increased in their agreement with sharing information openly with parents, validating statements about parents, valuing psychotropic medication for children and adolescents, and giving explicit instructions about ways to cope with their children's behavior.

The promising practice of family members serving as educators and consultants is also being implemented in North Carolina, at East Carolina University (Osher et al., 1999). In 1997, family members who helped in the planning and implementation of a Center for Mental Health Services grant joined together to create a family-run organization called WE CARE Federation of Families for Children's Mental Health. WE CARE-FFCMH partnered with East Carolina University's Social Sciences Training Consortium (SSTC) to offer pre-service and in-service training. The SSTC is a partnership among faculty in the departments/programs of Marriage and Family Therapy, Nursing, Psychiatry, Psychology, Recreational Therapy, and Social Work. The SSTC integrates system of care principles into graduate and undergraduate curricula, and ensures a family voice and presence in the classes through a contract with WE CARE-FFCMH.

Four faculty members of the SSTC created an interdisciplinary course called *Interdisciplinary Practice: Services for Children with Serious Emotional Disorders and Their Families*. The course is co-taught by all four-faculty members and family members. Family members who teach this course, and guest lecture in other university courses are called Parents in Residence (PIR). Having PIR's on the university campus helped integrate a parent's perspective into the curriculum as this course was being developed.

Parents in Residence had a significant impact on the students as well as the faculty. The students, most of whom were already working in the field with families, gained a more positive attitude about parent involvement, and became less blaming of families. These students got a real feel of how important their collaboration with other agency providers, extended family members, and community helpers were to the success of the child and family.

The impact on the faculty was just as critical. The faculty were able to build positive relationships with family members as they worked so closely together to develop and teach the course. These faculty began to invite family members to guest lecture in several other courses they taught at the university. There were many opportunities for them to witness first hand how often crisis happened with these families. These faculty members had a wealth of knowledge in their area of expertise, and years of experience serving families. Very often in a meeting called to plan for the class, a brain storming session happened to give support to one of the family members in crisis with their child. On more than one occasion, faculty members attended school meetings about a parent's child. Faculty members also served as support to the family at an individual service team meeting where agency providers, schools and community supports gathered to come up with a plan to best meet the need of that particular child and family.

Although the impact on students and faculty was great, the impact on the family members teaching the classes was even greater. The parents were scared and intimidated about being on a college campus, and teaching students who already had undergraduate degrees or who already worked in the system. The family members were pleasantly surprised at how well they were received by the students and the faculty. Family members were empowered as their perspectives about working with providers and dealing with agencies was validated. Family members were assured that these students would think differently about working with families with children with severe emotional and mental challenges. The students would understand the tremendous struggle around getting the needed services and supports, and become advocates themselves for families.

Family members bring two very unique and important perspectives: one of caregivers rearing a special needs child, and one as consumers trying to navigate many systems, agencies and community supports to get needed services. It is of grave importance that anyone working, or preparing to work, with these families learns to listen to their perspectives.

FAMILY MEMBERS AS ADVOCATES AND POLICY MAKERS

Families raising children with serious emotional and mental health challenges have struggled for years to empower themselves to work within Systems of Care to get the support and services for their child and family. Family members play an important role as local, statewide and national advocates and policy makers. Families have always been advocates for their own children. There have been many advocacy and support groups in the country that addressed mental retardation, developmental disability, and physical disabilities for quite some time. It has been in the last decade that family members of children with serious emotional disturbances have organized to gain support and to advocate on behalf of these children.

A national organization with over one hundred chapters across the country called the Federation of Families for Children's Mental Health was formed to support this population of families. This national parent-run organization focuses on the needs of children and youth with emotional, behavioral, or mental disorders and their families. The national Federation, as well as its many affiliates across the country, holds these principles to be true about children and youth with emotional, behavioral or mental health disorders. These children . . .

- Have unique needs that require individualized services
- Must be respected for their rights, preferences, values, strengths, culture and racial backgrounds
- Are entitled to full citizenship in their community
- Must receive what is necessary to achieve their full potential
- Belong with families and need enduring relationships with adults
- Make positive contributions to their families

- Must receive supports necessary to remain with their families; out-of-home placements must be considered as a last resort (Federation of Families for Children's Mental Health, n.d.).

The Federation contends that when children cannot remain with their families, out-of-home placement must be viewed as temporary and as an extension of the family. This treatment must be available close to the child's home and family members must be involved in all decisions regarding their child.

Providers such as social workers, therapists, teachers have all been advocates on behalf of children with serious emotional disturbances. Although their advocacy efforts have had some impact, family members have a long term obligation, as well as an emotional investment in their children's well being, that goes far beyond that of a hired provider. In most cases, family members are with the child for the long haul, while providers come and go (Friesen & Huff, 1990). Family members have first hand experience that make then credible advocates for systems change.

One example of how family members influenced policy through effective advocacy was with public schools' special education legislation. This legislation mandated parent involvement in the development of the Individualized Education Plan (IEP) (Public Law 94-142). Many family members wrote letters, called their legislators, and spoke with local school members about family involvement in the special education program. This greatly influenced the reauthorization of the Individuals with Disabilities Education Act of 1990 (PL 101-476). The Parent Advocacy Center for Education Rights (PACER Center) offers technical assistance to parent centers, disseminates information, and serves as a resource to professionals in the fields of education, health, and human services. It can be reached on the Internet (*www.pacer.org*).

All across the country, family members serve on boards and committees that shape and govern services for children with serious emotional disturbances. In 1986 Congress mandated family participation in developing state mental health plans (State Mental Health Services Comprehensive Plan, Public Law 99-660). The Alcohol, Drug Abuse, and Mental Health Administration Reorganization Act (Public Law 102-321) continues this mandate today (Family Participation in Policymaking, 1998). Family members chair client rights committees, serve as board of director members for major mental health agencies, and school boards. These family members are able to speak to such issues as:

- The lack of services
- The need for respite services
- Better parent-professional collaboration

- The lack of education and understanding about children's mental health issues
- The lack of family support
- Families' lack of knowledge on agencies' missions
- Issues around out-of-home foster or residential placements
- The challenge in getting different agency providers to collaborate around one family.

In the state of North Carolina, in the implementation of comprehensive community based service grants for families of children with serious emotional disturbances, family members were involved at every level of planning, implementation and evaluation. Families were represented on all committees, and served as advocates, trainers, data collectors, and in some cases, case managers. Families serving in these roles fostered relationship building between parents and providers (Simpson et al., 1999).

There were some instances in which providers asked families to help on policy issues within their agencies. Often, providers have legal restraints, or fear repercussion from supervisors if they speak out on behalf of a family member who is not receiving appropriate services. One such example was in a rural county in North Carolina. The mental health area program had experienced budget cuts. In the attempt to give employees a 3% raise, a plan was developed to close three satellite mental health clinics. These satellite clinics were very convenient to families living in the rural portion of the county, in which transportation is a huge issue. Many families would not be able to travel to the main mental health office, meaning their children would not get the services they needed. This change would also cost some workers their jobs, and the level of services would diminish.

Mental health providers approached a local family-run organization in the community, and asked them to advocate against closing the satellite clinics. Mental health center employees were willing to pass up the 3% raise so that co-workers would not lose their jobs, and the children would still get the services needed in their community. The family organization contacted the families that would most be affected by the change and asked them to attend the next board meeting where the issue would be up for vote. The local media were invited also. On the day of the board meeting, there was standing room only. Family members told the board how important the satellite clinics were, and also explained the transportation issues. The vote took place, and the clinics were saved (at least until the next round of deeper budget cuts).

When family members are invited and welcomed partners in the service delivery process for their children, they not only advocate for personal services and supports, but as policy makers, they provoke positive change in the delivery system. Social workers and many other service providers are accustomed to being advocates for families. The challenge is to partner with families to be more effective advocates. In order to form this partnership providers must also be willing to become change agents. This change must include the way family members are viewed by providers. We must not see them as part of the problem, but as experts on their own children. No matter what challenges the family may have, all families have strengths. The provider must look for these strengths and use them as a tool in reaching the family.

FAMILY MEMBERS AS EVALUATORS AND RESEARCHERS

Increasingly, family members are assuming active roles in the area of children's mental health research and evaluation. This involvement parallels the general shift toward including consumers and family members in all aspects of planning and evaluation of services, but also reflects recognition by researchers and evaluators of some unique advantages to be gained from family member participation in research activities. These advantages include identification of more meaningful and relevant research questions, higher quality data collection, and caregiver empowerment (Barnes, 1995; Carpenter, 1997, Koroloff & Friesen, 1997; Turnbull, Friesen, & Ramirez, 1998).

Family members are engaged in a number of expanded roles in research and evaluation. At the child and family level, family members participate in the evaluation of the services that they and their children receive both through the increased use of a variety of quality control and satisfaction measures (Anderson, Rivera, & Kutash, 1998), and through the review of processes and outcome findings related to their service packages. At the organizational and system levels, family members are engaged as advisors and members of site review teams for large scale evaluations (Stroul, McCormack, & Zaro, 1996), as members of evaluation teams as evaluation planners and data collectors, as authors of research reports, and as peer reviewers in federal grant processes.

A number of federal agencies actively encourage grantees to include consumers and family members in research and evaluation. For example, the National Institute on Disability and Rehabilitation Research supports a participatory action research model (Fenton, Batavia, & Roody, 1993), and the Center for Mental Health Services includes specific requirements for consumer and family involvement in its grant announcements.

Until recently family members who did not have formal training gained their research knowledge primarily through on-the-job experience. Now, however, more formal materials (Karp & Nolte, 1990; Nicholson & Robinson, 1996) and evaluation training is available for family members. For example, the Federation of Families for Children's Mental Health has developed training modules to provide an introduction to evaluation goals and concepts (Level I), and to prepare family members with skills to serve as full members of evaluation teams (Level II). A third level of evaluation training is envisioned as preparing family members to assume leadership in the research and evaluation process through identifying the research topic and playing a major role in the design, implementation, analysis, and interpretation phases of research endeavors (Federation of Families for Children's Mental Health, 1999; Turnbull et al., 1998).

Effectively implementing this relatively new role for families involves challenges for family members and for the direct service workers and evaluators working with them. At the individual child and family level the use of feedback to treatment teams about results obtained through evaluation requires attention to issues of trust, communication, and confidentiality. At the systems level, evaluators and family members must also establish trust, learn how to communicate about complicated concepts, and establish clear agreements about decision making, i.e., what the concept of partnership means in this context (Turnbull et al., 1998).

SUGGESTIONS FOR SERVICE PROVIDERS AND EDUCATORS

The empowering outcomes of participatory action research (Turnbull et al., 1998) apply to many of the expanded family roles identified and discussed here: helping family members take action to get what they want and need; increasing the opportunities of family members to contribute and offer input; promoting opportunities for researchers (and service providers) to have significant opportunities to learn about the realities of families' lives and the nature of family support; and expanding the collective power of families, service providers, and researchers through their collaboration with each other. Most significantly, this requires "a fundamental change in the nature of the relationship between professionals and the families served–from a relationship clearly marked by boundaries such as 'therapist' and 'client' to a relationship based on partnership and the mutual collaboration of the skills, knowledge, and experiences of each" (Hunter & Friesen, 1996, p. 19). Following are suggestions for service providers, and those who educate and train them, for putting this partnership ideal into practice.

1. "Listen carefully to what parents tell you and be open to new perspectives" (Friesen & Huff, 1990). Parents have reported that professionals often appear to agree or understand, but then ignore or distort parent input. Service providers can also learn about the issues and concerns of parents and siblings, and the family experience of mental illness, through continuing education programs, publications, and initiatives of such groups as national professional organizations and family organizations (Marsh & Johnson, 1997). They can ask family members to

speak to professional groups, as well as include them in pre-service and in-service educational programs.

2. In accordance with general psychotherapy literature, the quality of the working alliance with family members is a central consideration. Promoting "a respectful and empathic attitude toward families, an understanding of their phenomenological reality, an effort to meet their expressed needs, and a goal of family empowerment" are likely to develop a constructive alliance (Marsh & Johnson, 1997, p. 236). In a study on collaboration between social workers and families of persons with mental illness, DeChillo (1993) found that the strongest predictor of collaboration was the provider's attitude toward family involvement in the client's treatment. The degree of collaboration was important, as it was related not only to the family's satisfaction with the social work services received, but also with the degree of family involvement in the discharge-planning process (which has been found to have implications for better post-discharge functioning and lower likelihood of relapse).
3. "Be a resource to parents" (Friesen & Huff, 1990; Marsh & Johnson, 1997). Provide information, answer questions, and share your professional expertise with individuals and family groups (as in informing about mental illnesses and their treatment, teaching skills for coping, helping analyze a policy or piece of legislation). Educate regarding potential benefits, risks, costs, and research support for the effectiveness of services. Professionals can often offer practical support: media contacts, mailing lists, help preparing and printing newsletters, postage, and meeting space.
4. Service providers can help parents develop as advocates. Providers can inform parents of training opportunities, conferences and workshops, and help provide financial support and transportation for their attendance (Friesen & Huff, 1990; Friesen & Osher, 1996). When parents volunteer to attend meetings or assist with advocacy, professionals should be sensitive to the parents' other family and work obligations, as well as the logistics of travel and lodging expense, meeting, and arrangements for child care. Professionals also need to be aware that encouraging parents to be informed and assertive can result in conflict and criticism for the professionals; parents may become frustrated and angry when they become aware of the discrepancies between ideal and available services. Helping to negotiate conflict and focusing on the overall goals of improving services and quality of life are helpful. Service providers may also need to be candid about their own limitations, barriers to change, and the difference between their private opinions and the stance of their agency (Friesen & Huff, 1990).

5. Service providers and educators can insist on family participation in meetings, task forces, and organizational operations. They can ask, "Where are the family members?" and help locate family members to participate (Friesen & Huff, 1990).

Recognition of the seven expanded family roles described here may help service providers be better prepared to work collaboratively with families and family organizations, and to become aware of the accomplishments that may be achieved through such collaboration. The family member of our writing team offers our last words, "Families should not be viewed just as complainers, because often times the services rendered are not meeting the needs of the family. When families feel empowered enough to share what is or is not working for their family, positive changes can be made in the services, thus leading to better outcomes. Realize that family members are your greatest resource in serving the children within your agency."

REFERENCES

Angold, A., Messer, S. C., Stangl, D., Farmer, E. M. Z., Costello, E. J., & Burns, B. J. (1998). Perceived parental burden and service use for child and adolescent psychiatric disorders. *American Journal of Public Health, 88*, 75-80.

Anderson, J. A., Rivera, V. B., & Kutash, K. (1998). Measuring consumer satisfaction with children's mental health services (pp. 455-481). In M.H. Epstein, K. Kutash, & A. Duchnowski (Eds.), *Outcomes for children and youth with emotional and behavioral disorders and their families: Programs and evaluation best practices*. Austin, TX: Pro-Ed.

Barnes, J. (1995). *Family collaboration in systems evaluation.* TA Brief, 1 (1). Boston, MA: Center for the Evaluation of Children's Mental Health Systems, Judge Baker Children's Center.

Brannan, A. M., Heflinger, C. A. & Bickman, L. (1997). The caregiver strain questionnaire: Measuring the impact on the family of living with a child with serious emotional disturbance. *Journal of Emotional and Behavioral Disorders, 5*(4), 212-222.

Burchard, J. D. & Clarke, R. T. (1990). The role of individualized care in a service delivery system for children and adolescents with severely maladjusted behavior. *The Journal of Mental Health Administration, 17*(1), 48-60.

Burns, B. J. & Goldman, S. K. (Eds.) (1999). *Promising practices in wraparound for children with serious emotional disturbance and their families.* Systems of Care: Promising Practices in Children's Mental Health, 1998 Series, Volume IV. Washington, DC: Center for Effective Collaboration and Practice, American Institutes for Research.

Carpenter, B. (1997). Empowering parents: The use of the parent as researcher paradigm in early intervention. *Journal of Child and Family Studies, 6*(4), 391-398.

Center for Mental Health Services. (1996). Prevalence of serious emotional disturbance in children and adolescents. *Mental Health, United States, 1996.* Center for Mental Health Services, Substance Abuse and Mental Health Services Administration, U.S. Department of Health and Human Services.

Cournoyer, D. E. & Johnson, H. C. (1991). Measuring parents' perceptions of mental health professionals. *Research on Social Work Practice, 1*(4), 399-415.

DeChillo, N. (1993). Collaboration between social workers and families of patients with mental illness. *Families in Society: The Journal of Contemporary Human Services, 74*(2), 104-114.

DeChillo, N., Koren, P. E. & Schultze, K. H. (1994). From paternalism to partnership: Family and professional collaboration in children's mental health. *American Journal of Orthopsychiatry, 64*, 564-576.

Dunlap, K. M. (1997). Family empowerment: One outcome of cooperative preschool education. *Child Welfare, 76*(4), 501-518.

Erchul, W. P., & Raven, B. H. (1997). Social power in school consultation: A contemporary view of French and Raven's bases of power model. *Journal of School Psychology, 35*(2), 137-171.

Family Participation in Policymaking. (1998). *Focal Point: A National Bulletin on Family Support & Children's Mental Health, 12*(1), 1-5.

Farmer, E. M. Z., Burns, B. J., Angold, A., & Costello, E. (1997). Impact of children's mental health problems on families: Relationships with service use. *Journal of Emotional and Behavioral Disorders, 5*(4), 230-238.

Federation of Families for Children's Mental Health. (n.d.). A parent-run organization focused on the needs of children and youth with emotional, behavioral, or mental disorders and their families. (pamphlet) 1101 King Street, Suite 420, Alexandria, VA 22314.

Federation of Families for Children's Mental Health (1999). *The world of evaluation: How to make it yours.* Alexandria, VA: Federation of Families for Children's Mental Health.

Fenton, J., Batavia, A. & Roody, D. S. (1993). *Proposed Policy Statement for NIDRR on Constituency-Oriented Research and Dissemination (CORD).* Washington, D.C.: National Institute on Disability and Rehabilitation Research, U.S. Department of Education.

Friesen, B. J. & Huff, B. (1990). Parents and professionals as advocacy partners. In *Preventing School Failure* (formerly *The Pointer*), *34*(3), 31-35.

Friesen, B. J. & Huff, B. (1996). Family perspectives on systems of care. In B.A. Stroul (Ed.), *Children's mental health: Creating systems of care in a changing society*, (pp. 41-67). Baltimore: Brookes.

Friesen, B. J., Koren, P.E., & Koroloff, N. M. (1992). How parents view professional behaviors: A cross-professional analysis. *Journal of Child and Family Studies, 1*(2), 209-231.

Friesen, B. J. & Osher, T. W. (1996). Involving families in change: challenges and opportunities (pp. 187-207). In R. J. Illback & C. M. Nelson (Eds.), *Emerging school-based approaches for children with emotional and behavioral problems: Research and practice in service integration.* New York: The Haworth Press, Inc.

Friesen, B. J. & Stephens, B. (1998). Expanding family roles in the system of care:

Research and practice. In M. H. Epstein, K. Kutash, & A. Duchnowski (Eds.). *Outcomes for children and youth with emotional and behavioral disorders and their families: Programs and evaluation best practices*, (pp. 231-259). Austin, TX: PRO-ED.

Friesen, B. J. & Wahlers, D. (1993). Respect and real help: Family support and children's mental health. *Journal of Emotional & Behavioral Problems, 2*(4), 12-15.

Hasenfeld, Y. (1987). Power in social work practice. *Social Service Review, 61*(3), 467-483.

Heflinger, C. A. & Bickman, L. (1996). Family empowerment: A conceptual model for promoting parent-professional partnership (pp. 96-112). In C. A. Heflinger and C. T. Nixon (Eds.), *Families and the mental health system for children and adolescents: Policy, services, and research.* Thousand Oaks, CA: Sage.

Hunter, R. W. & Friesen, B. J. (1996). Family-centered services for children with emotional, behavioral, and mental disorders (pp. 18-37). In C. A. Heflinger & C. T. Nixon (Eds.), *Families and the mental health system for children and adolescents: Policy, services, and research.* Thousand Oaks, CA: Sage.

Ignelzi, S. & Dague, B. (1995). Parents as case managers (pp. 327-336). In B. J. Friesen & J. Poertner, (Eds.), *From case management to service coordination for children with emotional, behavioral, or mental disorders: Building on family strengths.* Baltimore, MD: Brookes.

Jivanjee, R. R. & Friesen, B. J. (1997). Shared expertise: Family participation in interprofessional training. *Journal of Emotional and Behavioral Disorders, 5*(4), 205-211.

Johnson, D. L. (1994). Current issues in family research: Can the burden of mental illness be relieved? (pp. 309-328). In H. P. Lefley & M. Wasow (Eds.), *Helping families cope with mental illness.* USA: Harwood.

Johnson, H. C. (in press). The Power of Parent-Professor Partnerships. In C. Liberton, C. Newman, K. Kutash, & R. Friedman, (Eds.), The 13th Annual Research Conference Proceedings, A System of Care for Children's Mental Health: Expanding the Research Base (March 2000). Tampa, FL: University of South Florida, The Louis de la Parte Florida Mental Health Institute, Research and Training Center for Children's Mental Health.

Johnson, H. C., Cournoyer, D. E. & Fisher, G. A. (1994). Measuring worker cognitions about parents of children with mental and emotional disabilities. *Journal of Emotional and Behavioral Disorders, 2*(2), 99-108.

Karp, N. & Nolte, C. (1990). *Grant writer's guide.* Washington, DC: The National Institute on Disability and Rehabilitation Research, Office of Special Education and Rehabilitative Services, U.S. Department of Education.

Koroloff, N. M., Elliott, D. J., Koren, P. E., & Friesen, B. J. (1996). Linking low-income families to children's mental health services: An outcome study. *Journal of Emotional and Behavioral Disorders, 4*, 2-11.

Koroloff, N. M. & Friesen, B. J. (1997). Challenges in conducting family-centered mental health services research. *Journal of Emotional and Behavioral Disorders, 5*(3), 130-37.

Koroloff, N. M., Friesen, B. J., Reilly, L., Rinkin, J. (1996). The role of family members in systems of care (pp. 409-425). In B. A. Stroul (Ed.), *Children's mental health: Creating systems of care in a changing society.* Baltimore, MD: Brookes.

Lee, J. A. B. (1994). The empowerment approach: A conceptual framework (pp. 11-38). In J. A. Lee (Ed.), *The empowerment approach to social work practice.* New York: Columbia University Press.

Marsh, D. T. (1996). Families of children and adolescents with serious emotional disturbance: Innovations in theory, research, and practice (pp. 75-95). In C. A. Heflinger & C. T. Nixon (Eds.), *Families and the mental health system for children and adolescents: Policy, services, and research.* Thousand Oaks, CA: Sage.

Marsh, D. T. & Johnson, D. L. (1997). The family experience of mental illness: Implications for intervention. *Professional Psychology: Research and Practice, 28,* 229-237.

Moore-Kirkland, J. (1981). Mobilizing motivation: From theory to practice. In A. N. Maluccio (Ed.), *Promoting Competence in Clients,* pp. 27-54. New York: Free Press.

Nicholson, J. & Robinson, G. (1996). *A guide for evaluating consumer satisfaction with children and adolescent mental health services.* Boston, MA: Center for the Evaluation of Children's Mental Health Systems, Judge Baker Children's Center.

Osher, T. W., Defur, E., Nava, C., Spencer, S., & Toth-Dennis, D. (1999). New roles for families in systems of care. In *Systems of Care: Promising Practices in Children's Mental Health 1998 Series, Volume 1.* Washington, D.C.: Center for Effective Collaboration and Practice, American Institutes for Research.

Pinderhughes, E. (1995). Empowering diverse populations: Family practice in the 21st century. *Families in Society, 76*(3), 131-140.

Reisser, G. G. & Schorske, B. J. (1994). Relationships between family caregivers and mental health professionals: The American experience (pp. 3-26). In H. P. Lefley & M. Wasow (Eds.), *Helping families cope with mental illness,* USA: Harwood.

Sakwa, D. & Ireys, H. T. (1998, June). Parent Connections: A family-professional collaboration for youth with serious emotional disorders. Workshop conducted at the meeting, The 11th Annual Research Conference, A System of Care for Children's Mental Health: Expanding the Research Base, Orlando, FL.

Saleeby, D. (1996). The strengths perspective in social work practice: Extensions and cautions. *Social Work, 41*(3), 296-305.

Simpson, J. S., Koroloff, N., Friesen, B. F., & Gac, J. (1999). *Promising practices in family-provider collaboration.* System of Care: Promising Practices in Children's Mental Health, 1998 Series, Volume II. Washington, D.C.: Center for Effective Collaboration and Practice, American Institutes for Research.

Stroul, B. A. & Friedman, R. M. (1996). The system of care concept and philosophy (pp. 3-21). In B. A. Stroul (Ed.), *Children's mental health: Creating systems of care in a changing society.* Baltimore, MD: Brookes.

Stroul, B. A., Friedman, R. M., Hernandez, M. Roebuck, L. Lourie, I. S., & Koyanagi, C. (1996). Conclusion: Systems of care in the future. In B. A. Stroul (Ed.). *Children's mental health: Creating systems of care in a changing society.* Baltimore, MD: Brookes, p. 591-612.

Stroul, B. A., McCormack, M., & Zaro, S. M. (1996). Measuring outcomes in systems of care. In B.A. Stroul (Ed.), *Children's mental health services: Creating systems of care in a changing society* (pp. 313-336). Baltimore: Brookes.

Tannen, N. (1996). *Families at the center of the development of a system of care.* Washington, DC: National Technical Assistance Center for Children's Mental Health, Georgetown University.

Thomas, N. E. & Friesen, B. J. (Eds.) (1990). *Next Steps: Conference Proceedings.* Portland, OR: Research and Training Center on Family Support and Children's Mental Health, Portland State University.

Turnbull, A. P., Friesen, B. J., & Ramirez, C. (1998). Participatory action research as a model for conducting family research. *The Journal of the Association for Persons with Severe Handicaps*, 23(3), 178-188.

VanDenBerg, J. & Grealish, M. (1996). Individualized services and supports through the wraparound process: Philosophy and procedures. *Journal of Child and Family Studies*, *5*(1), 7-21.

Williams-Murphy, T., DeChillo, N., Koren, P. E., & Hunter, R. (1994). *Family/professional collaboration: The perspectives of those who have tried.* Portland, OR: Portland State University, Research and Training Center on Family Support and Children's Mental Health.

Yatchmenoff, D. K., Koren, P. E., Friesen, B. J., Gordon, L. J., & Kinney, R. F. (1998). Enrichment and stress in families caring for a child with a serious emotional disorder. *Journal of Child and Family Studies*, *7*(2), 129-145.

In Quest of an Interdisciplinary Helping Process Framework for Collaborative Practice in Systems of Care

John Y. Powell, PhD
Ashton Privette, MSW
Scott D. Miller, PhD
James K. Whittaker, PhD

SUMMARY. The "'Heart and Soul of Change': Therapies for a New Century" interdisciplinary symposium developed from a personal dream. The dream grew out of a collaborative, community-wide "sys-

---

John Y. Powell is Professor Emeritus and Ashton Privette is a graduate student, School of Social Work and Criminal Justice Studies, East Carolina University. Scott D. Miller is Psychologist, Family Therapist and Co-Founder, Institute for the Study of Therapeutic Change, Chicago, IL. James K. Whittaker is Professor, School of Social Work, University of Washington, Seattle, WA.

Address correspondence to: John Y. Powell, School of Social Work and Criminal Justice Studies, Ragsdale Hall, East Carolina University, Greenville, NC 27858-4353 (E-mail: powellj@mail.ecu.edu).

The authors express appreciation to Ms. Traci Lynch for assistance in manuscript preparation.

Preparation of the manuscript was funded in part through a contract with the North Carolina Division of Mental Health, Developmental Disabilities and Substance Abuse Services, Child and Family Services, as a component of the System of Care: Training and Curriculum Development Project, funded by a grant from the Center for Mental Health Services.

[Haworth co-indexing entry note]: "In Quest of an Interdisciplinary Helping Process Framework for Collaborative Practice in Systems of Care." Powell, John Y. et al. Co-published simultaneously in *Journal of Family Social Work* (The Haworth Social Work Practice Press, an imprint of The Haworth Press, Inc.) Vol. 5, No. 3, 2001, pp. 25-34; and: *Child Mental Health: Exploring Systems of Care in the New Millennium* (ed: David A. Dosser, Jr. et al.) The Haworth Social Work Practice Press, an imprint of The Haworth Press, Inc., 2001, pp. 25-34. Single or multiple copies of this article are available for a fee from The Haworth Document Delivery Service [1-800-342-9678, 9:00 a.m. - 5:00 p.m. (EST). E-mail address: getinfo@haworth pressinc. com].

© 2001 by The Haworth Press, Inc. All rights reserved.

tem of care" project which helped children with serious emotional disturbances and their families receive comprehensive services. To support the community's system of care project, East Carolina University assembled a team of faculty from a cross-section of professional "helping" disciplines. A core faculty group accepted the responsibility of developing a curriculum and teaching an interdisciplinary, collaborative practice course. They soon realized that professional literature lacked conceptual frameworks that could guide professionals from various disciplines who practice in "systems of care" or use "wraparound" techniques. In such settings, professionals are expected to collaborate together and be "partners with families." As a result, they decided to bring together Dr. Scott D. Miller and Dr. James K. Whittaker to lead a symposium to help build a unifying framework for collaborative, interdisciplinary practice. Using a personal format, this essay tells how the symposium developed, and it gives a brief overview of its presentations. Finally it concludes with several post-symposium questions addressed to Dr. Miller and Dr. Whittaker that help further develop a framework for interdisciplinary, collaborative practice. This information will be of use to serve providers as they attempt to develop a framework for their work. Further, it is expected that the questions addressed in this essay are questions that all service providers need to consider as they work collaboratively with children and families. *[Article copies available for a fee from The Haworth Document Delivery Service: 1-800-342-9678. E-mail address: <getinfo@haworthpressinc.com> Website: <http://www.HaworthPress.com> © 2001 by The Haworth Press, Inc. All rights reserved.]*

KEYWORDS. Helping process, collaborative practice, therapy, elements of therapy, person/environment practice, system of care, children with serious emotional disturbances

INTRODUCTION

I began my professional career in a children's residential center and continued to work in residential treatment settings until joining the faculty of ECU in 1987. In residential settings, collaboration and interdisciplinary practice are essential if service providers desire to create truly therapeutic environments for children and youth with serious emotional disturbances (Powers, 1980). Additionally, research indicates that gains made by children while in residential treatment settings tend to erode unless agencies help create linkages between the residential staff and the children's families and communities (for example see Allerhand, Weber & Haug, 1966). Later Whittaker (1979) concluded that parents need to be partners with residential agencies to maximize the potential of placements.

In residential treatment settings, staff routinely work as interdisciplinary teams in concert with the children's families and referring professionals. Assuming that interdisciplinary cooperation was widely accepted, I was surprised and dismayed upon becoming a professor of Social Work to discover how separate and "turf oriented" various professional disciplines (including my own) had become in academia.

I, therefore, have sought ways to promote collaboration and interdisciplinary practice and research at ECU. Four colleagues and I developed a curriculum for and began to teach an interdisciplinary, collaborative practice course that was based on "system of care" and "wraparound" principles (Handron, Dosser, McCammon, & Powell, 1998; Powell, Handron, Dosser, McCammon, Temkin & Kaufman, 1999). We found some literature pertaining to systems of care and collaborative practice underpinnings to guide system of care practice with children and families coping with serious emotional disturbances. For example, one can locate texts that suggest ways that professionals can collaborate (Seaburn, Lorenz, Gunn, Gawinski, & Mauksch, 1996) or books that give an overview of the development of systems of care (Stroul, 1996), but little attention has been given to uniting therapeutic techniques, and the theoretical notions that spawned them, with practice realities. How might a psychiatrist, a mental health nurse practitioner, a family therapist, a psychologist, a social worker, a school guidance counselor, and a parent embark upon a therapeutic process together with one person being guided by a behavioral approach, another by a belief that physiological influences are paramount, yet another believing that change is based on cognitive reframing, and at the same time with a parent who feels that she or he is being blamed for the child's emotional disturbance? How might a parent be a colleague, and at the same time be encouraged to change his or her behavior? Is there a common, non-blaming therapeutic language that might be used by professionals and families alike that could promote collaboration and partnership?

With such thoughts in mind, in the Spring of 1999, I attended a conference in San Francisco and heard a thought provoking presentation by Dr. James K. Whittaker and colleagues that was based upon their book, *Person-Environment Practice: The Social Ecology of Interpersonal Helping* (Kemp, Whittaker, & Tracy, 1997). Later that evening, I flew across the continent to North Carolina to receive an award at a family therapy conference. The conference's featured speaker was Dr. Scott D. Miller who shared findings from the *Heart & Soul of Change: What Works in Therapy* (Hubble, Dixon, & Miller, 1999). As I reflected upon the presentations, I began to believe that the two speakers should be brought together in an academic symposium to help develop a process framework for interdisciplinary, collaborative practice with families who have children with serious emotional disturbances. Thus a symposium was held on February 24 and 25, 2000, at East Carolina University entitled "Heart and Soul of Change: Therapies for a New Century."

Summaries of the Presentations

With the symposium we hoped to lay a foundation for "system of care" practice by various disciplines, and sought to promote a sense of partnership between professionals and consumers. Ms. Sandra Spencer introduced this concept by opening the symposium from a consumer/family's perspective as she told of the struggles that families face in receiving appropriate treatment for their children with serious emotional disturbances (see Spencer & Powell, 2000). Following this introduction, the featured speakers, Dr. Scott Miller and Dr. James Whittaker, provided an interesting combination as they interplayed their practice, scholarly and research experiences with each other and the audience.

Dr. Scott Miller is well known as an author, psychologist, family therapist and co-founder of the Institute for the Study of Therapeutic Change in Chicago. Dr. Miller and his colleagues have analyzed successful psychotherapeutic research studies, and they believe that the components of therapeutic success can be roughly classified into four categories: "therapeutic relationship, 30%," "creating hope and expectancy, 15%," "therapeutic technique, 15%," and "extratherapeutic factors, 40%." The latter category, "extratherapeutic factors," is related to the everyday events in people's lives, and Dr. Miller and his colleagues contend that what happens outside the therapy session, these "extratherapeutic factors," are extremely important. He argued that current university training for mental health professionals tends to emphasize only 15% of outcome success, i.e., therapeutic technique. Dr. Miller observed: "Given the clear demonstrations from research that there is little appreciable difference in outcome among the various therapy models, it is puzzling that they remain the centerpiece of so much graduate professional training. How can something that makes so little difference continue to dominate professional discussion?"

Dr. James K. Whittaker, Professor of Social Work at the University of Washington at Seattle, is truly a "scholar in practice" as he has related his extensive professional writings (eight books and scores of articles) to practice realities. For example, he began his career in a residential treatment setting, and he and his colleagues turned the agency's staff training manual into a classic book, *The Other Twenty-Three Hours: Child Care Work in a Therapeutic Environment* (Trieschman, Whittaker & Bendtro, (1969). In *Person-Environment-Practice*, Dr. Whittaker and his co-authors have pioneered concepts and practice strategies which seek to help people enrich, expand and better fit into their natural environments (Kemp, Whittaker, & Tracy, 1997).

During the "Heart and Soul of Change" symposium, Dr. Whittaker emphasized that we must continually "rethink the role of 'environment' in interpersonal practice" using a research and development approach, and he shared the concepts, value bases and essential components of person-environment practice. These interventions capitalize on helping people use naturally occurring and intentionally developed environmental resources, such as better using and expanding their social support networks. Dr. Whittaker strongly believes that professionals and consumers share common human needs and problems. He noted: "We begin each foray into the practice arena recalling that, save for the vagaries of birth, errant biology, class and status, or simply circumstance, we are all but a step away from the 'other' human beings who are our 'needy' or 'at-risk' clients. In the final analysis it is not 'us' and 'them'; it is all of us together."

The presentations were complementary to many systems of care practice concepts. Both speakers emphasized the significance of relationship development and the sense of partnership between the client and the therapist as well as the importance of building on clients' strengths. For example, Dr. Miller used a videotape of a therapy session to point out the importance of a father attributing changes in his son's behavior to the son, not to the therapeutic boot camp he had attended. He gave the son credit for deciding to make positive behavioral changes, which focused on the son's strengths, and the father avoided simply giving credit to the boot camp, which only helped facilitate the changes.

In addition to Dr. Miller's presentation, his book, *Heart & Soul of Change: What Works in Therapy* (1999) includes research findings to convey the importance of seeing that the methods or techniques used in therapy fit the client's expectations (or the client's theory of change). In particular, it was noted that practitioners should let clients drive the change process–as opposed to the usual way of having professionals choose particular techniques. Hope and expectancy factors were also emphasized by Dr. Miller and other symposium speakers as important elements of change.

The speakers also cautioned against relying on the traditional hierarchical boundaries that exist between providers and consumers as they may hinder partnership development. Questions arose as to what is therapy? Should a client's life events and personal environment be considered "extratherapeutic factors"? Is person-environment practice also a therapeutic endeavor?

Dr. Miller suggested that his notions of "what works in therapy" not be thought of one dimensionally in which pieces are just put together, but to use the concepts as a prism or a new set of lens to look through. For example, isn't a behavioral intervention with a child more effective if a therapist relates well to the child and instills a sense of hope that the child's life can become more fulfilling in the future? In his *Heart & Soul of Change: What Works in Therapy* (1999) Miller suggests that "new" therapies many times are only a "repackaging" of essential therapeutic elements with a current spin that serves to increase consumer expectancy.

Dr. Whittaker's presentation was especially poignant as he used his experiences in residential settings to support systems of care notions. He was also able to move from the role of scholar to the personal role of a parent whose child has special needs-combining scholarly observations and personal examples. He made the distinction between what it felt like to be a provider of services and what it felt like to walk into a room as a client with helping professionals sitting on the other side of the desk. While he validated Dr. Miller's caution to avoid exaggerated claims of pharmaceutical manufacturers, he also recognized the importance of wisely using medication by describing how prescribed drugs in combination with cognitive and behavioral interventions had been helpful in his son's treatment. Dr. Whittaker questioned Dr. Miller's use of the term "extratherapeutic factors." Dr. Miller referred to this term as describing what occurs outside the office or outside the therapy session, but Dr. Whittaker asked if "therapy" should be so narrowly defined. Such questions are in line with current system of care practice as it can be viewed as a healing process that can occur at a community or organizational level as well as the family service level. System of care's broad definition of helping or therapy has helped to spawn new concepts and approaches such as "wraparound" services (Handron, Dosser, McCammon & Powell, 1998).

As readers can observe, the "Heart and Soul of Change: Therapies for a New Century" was a useful and informative event, and we are pleased that Dr. Miller and Dr. Whittaker have extended this learning experience by answering post-symposium questions. The questions were developed collaboratively by David Dosser, Dorothea Handron, Susan McCammon, John Powell and Sandra Spencer whose team teaches a graduate level course on interdisciplinary practice.

Questions for Dr. Whittaker and Dr. Miller:

1. *Theory and Technique*: Dr. Miller believes that only 15% of success with clients can be attributed to "therapeutic technique," and we feel that the term "technique" is not synonymous with "theory"-but students often confuse the two. In his writings, Dr. Whittaker has cited Kurt Lewin's idea "that there is nothing so valuable as a good theory." For example, a practitioner might be guided by systemic and ecological theoretical concepts, and yet use a variety of techniques. How might we teach students to differentiate between theory and technique-and at the same time unite the two in their practice?

Dr. Whittaker responded:

I wonder if the distinction is really between 'theory' and 'technique'? In my view, we obtain knowledge from many different sources to inform our practice. Three main sources are: (1) empirical research, (2) theory and (3) what might be thought of as the accumulated 'wisdom' of practitioners. Each of these knowledge sources has its strengths as well as its limits. For example, the research literature on 'family functioning' for many years lacked external validity with respect to African-Americans because of sample biases. Also, there are many areas where human services practitioners are asked to intervene where there does not yet exist a body of empirical evidence clearly favoring one intervention over another. In the case of theory, human services is replete with examples of untested theory as the sole source of practice knowledge: often with tragic results (recall the parent blaming that defined so much of clinical thinking in the 50s and 60s with respect to serious childhood disorders, for example). Similarly, with 'practice wisdom,' there are problems. When I entered the field in the 60s 'conventional' wisdom was that none of the following made good candidates for adoption: children over 1 year of age, single parents, childless couples, foster parents, gay or lesbian parents. Then along came special needs adoption, the practice of which has demonstrated that with the right supports, any of these sub-groups can participate in successful adoptions.

To me, theory/research/practice wisdom are inextricably linked. They are necessary, but not sufficient components of an overall knowledge base for practice. I believe the educational task is to help students identify the bases from which they are proceeding in a given situation and provide them the tools to critically compare and contrast differing knowledge sources for practice.

Dr. Miller responded:

For years, the practice of therapy has been guided by the formal theories of therapists. The result is a plethora of explanations for mental and emotional problems that number in the hundreds. Associated with each of these theories are usually a group of techniques believed to uniquely address the pathology as spelled out by the theory.

Our work emphasizes the informal theory of clients. That is, the ideas clients have about their problems, their causes and potential solutions, as well as their experiences with change in general. Rather than organizing treatment according to the therapist's theory, we recommend trying to understand and then follow the client's theory of change.

2. *What Is Therapy?*: How broadly should we define therapy? Should Person-Environment Practice be considered therapy, and how does

Person-Environment Practice fit with the concept of extratherapeutic factors? How can we help train future practitioners to unite and better apply the practice concepts presented at the symposium?

Dr. Whittaker responded:

To answer this question fully, one needs to be skilled in post-modern thinking and 'de-construction.' Since I possess neither the knowledge or the skill sets required, I'll simply say that the very language of the question suggests hierarchy: 'therapy' is the 'real stuff,' everything else is 'extratherapeutic' (read as "marginalized"). For me, the questions begin not with a professional role, but with differing client needs:

- What are they? How are they to be discerned (assessment)?
- What relationship ought to exist between "helpers" and "helped"?
- What things have people found helpful in professional behavior and how can these be replicated?
- What's our fundamental view of the relationship of person-to-environment and how is that view reflected in our interventions?

Dr. Miller responded:

The answer to this question is simple: Stop teaching students techniques and models of therapy. Experienced therapists appear to come to this way of thinking on their own after years of working in the field. The second step would be guiding training with valid and reliable feedback from clients regarding the process and outcome of treatment. Both of these would significantly decrease the competition among competing brands of therapy and increase the likelihood that therapists would organize their clinical work according to the common factors earlier in their career.

3. *In Quest of an Interdisciplinary Helping Process Framework for Collaborative Practice in Systems of Care*: As you reflect upon the title of this paper and the information shared at the symposium, what additional thoughts and suggestions would you now add?

Dr. Whittaker responded:

To me the most hopeful thing about the ECU symposium was the respectful way in which academic colleagues from a wide variety of disciplines came together with their practitioner counterparts to share knowledge, including differing perspectives, and struggle to identify some "better ways" of helping families and children with special needs.

To me the dominant themes from the audience, in other words, what I took away were: partnership, respect for difference, cultural competence, humility (in the face of sometimes overwhelming challenges) and a wonderful spirit of celebration.

I think the child and family field has much to learn from the ECU community partnership. It was a privilege to participate.

Dr. Miller responded:

In the early 1980s the president of the APA, Nicholas Cummings, began to sound the warning claxon regarding the changing mental health care market place. He advised therapists to set down their differences and work together to both accommodate and take the lead in addressing the coming changes. The response of professional mental health organizations and most providers was to ignore the warnings. The result is the crisis currently facing practitioners: eroding wages, diminished power to make clinical decisions, and poorer quality of mental healthcare for the average citizen. As far as I see it, the challenge of working together across disciplinary and theoretical lines remains. The work of my colleagues and I at the Institute for the Study of Therapeutic Change on the common factors is simply one attempt to facilitate a dialogue on what all do that works in treatment. This same ecumenical spirit was certainly reflected in the conference.

CONCLUSION

The quest for an "Interdisciplinary Helping Process Framework for Collaborative Practice in Systems of Care" is an emerging endeavor, and it will not be resolved easily or quickly. Rather, it is a process of discovery that will require clear thinking, careful research and the emergence of practice wisdom as families and professionals work respectfully together. It is hoped that this article may be useful in this quest.

REFERENCES

Allerhand, M.E., Weber, R.E., Haug, M. (1966). *Adaptation and adaptability: The Bellefaire follow-up study.* New York: Child Welfare League of America.

Handron, D.S., Dosser, D.A., Jr., McCammon, S.L. & Powell, J.Y. (1998). "Wrap-around" the wave of the future: Theoretical and practice implications for children with complex needs. *Journal of Family Nursing, 4*(1), 65-86.

Hubble, M.A., Dixon, B.L. & Miller, S.D. (1999). *Heart & soul of change: What works in therapy.* Washington: American Psychological Association.

Kemp, S.P., Whittaker, J.K. & Tracy, E.M. (1997). *Person-environment practice: The social ecology of interpersonal helping.* New York: Aldine de Gruyter.

Powell, J., Handron, D., Dosser, D., McCammon, S., Temkin, M., & Kaufman, M. (1999). Challenges of interdisciplinary collaboration: A faculty consortium's initial attempts to model collaborative practice. *Journal of Community Practice, 6*(2), 27-48.

Powers, D. (1980). *Creating environments for troubled children.* Chapel Hill: University of NC Press.

Seaburn, D.B., Lorenz, A.D., Gunn, W.B., Gawinski, B.A. & Mauksch, L.B. (1996). *Models of collaboration: A guide for mental health professionals working with health care practitioners.* New York: Basic Books.

Spencer, S. & Powell, J.Y. (2000). Family-centered practice in residential treatment settings: A parent's perspective. *Residential Treatment for Children & Youth, 17*(3), 33-43.

Stroul, B.A. (1996). *Children's mental health: Creating systems of care in a changing society.* Baltimore, MD: Brookes Publishing.

Trieschman, A.E., Whittaker, J.K., Brendtro, L.K. (1969). *The other twenty-three hours: Childcare work in a therapeutic milieu.* New York: Aldine de Gruyter.

Whittaker, J.K. (1997). *Caring for troubled children: Residential treatment in a community context.* New York: Aldine de Gruyter.

Words Can Be Powerful: Changing the Words of Helping to Enhance Systems of Care

Lessie L. Bass, DSW
David A. Dosser, Jr., PhD
John Y. Powell, PhD

SUMMARY. In this paper, the schema for family-centered practice is proposed as a tool that would make it easier for workers to practice according to system of care values and principles. The use of a system of care model of practice requires both providers and consumers of services to make a paradigm shift in their thinking about how assistance

---

Lessie L. Bass is Associate Professor and John Y. Powell is Professor Emeritus in the School of Social Work and Criminal Justice Studies, East Carolina University. David A. Dosser, Jr. is Director and Associate Professor, Marriage and Family Therapy Program, Department of Child Development and Family Relations, School of Human Environmental Sciences, East Carolina University.

Address correspondence to: Lessie L. Bass, DSW, Associate Professor, School of Social Work and Criminal Justice Studies, East Carolina University, Greenville, NC 27858 (E-mail: bassl@mail.ecu.edu).

Appreciation is expressed to Ms. Traci Lynch for assistance in manuscript preparation.

Preparation of the manuscript was funded in part through a contract with the North Carolina Division of Mental Health, Developmental Disabilities and Substance Abuse Services, Child and Family Services, as a component of the System of Care: Training and Curriculum Development Project, funded by a grant from the Center for Mental Health Services.

Portions of this article appeared earlier in an essay [Powell, J. Y. (1996) A schema for family-centered practice. *Families in Society, 17*(30), 446-448].

[Haworth co-indexing entry note]: "Words Can Be Powerful: Changing the Words of Helping to Enhance Systems of Care." Bass, Lessie L., David A. Dosser, Jr., and John Y. Powell. Co-published simultaneously in *Journal of Family Social Work* (The Haworth Social Work Practice Press, an imprint of The Haworth Press, Inc.) Vol. 5, No. 3, 2001, pp. 35-48; and: *Child Mental Health: Exploring Systems of Care in the New Millennium* (ed: David A. Dosser, Jr. et al.) The Haworth Social Work Practice Press, an imprint of The Haworth Press, Inc., 2001, pp. 35-48. Single or multiple copies of this article are available for a fee from The Haworth Document Delivery Service [1-800-342-9678, 9:00 a.m. - 5:00 p.m. (EST). E-mail address: getinfo@haworthpressinc.com].

© 2001 by The Haworth Press, Inc. All rights reserved.

is conveyed. The model emphasizes forging a partnership between service providers and consumers rather than founding the helping relationship on a more traditional hierarchical approach that places the provider in the role of expert. Unfortunately, much of the language used by the helping professions reinforces a more conventional provider-as-expert approach. To assist providers and consumers in making the necessary paradigm shift away from the provider-as-expert approach, the authors propose using a schema for family-centered practice (schema). The schema, comprised of six steps (Joining > Discovery > Changing > Celebrating > Separating > Reflection), promotes the use of a new user-friendly language format, which is consistent with system of care's thinking and practice focus on partnering consumers and service providers. The values of the schema as a tool for use in system of care work along with descriptions of the experiences of service providers and consumers in using the schema are included as are suggestions for its use. *[Article copies available for a fee from The Haworth Document Delivery Service: 1-800-342-9678. E-mail address: <getinfo@haworthpressinc.com> Website: <http://www.HaworthPress.com> © 2001 by The Haworth Press, Inc. All rights reserved.]*

KEYWORDS. Family support, family-centered, child-centered, schema, systems of care, partnership, collaboration

Words can be powerful. Words have been known to change an individual, a group, a family or an entire nation's future. Remember the words that Dr. Martin Luther King, Jr. delivered on the 28th of August 1963:

> I have a dream that one day this nation will rise up and live out the true meaning of its creed: "We hold these truths to be self-evident, that all men are created equal." And when this happens, when we allow freedom to ring, when we let it ring from every village and every hamlet, from every state and every city, we will be able to speed up that day when all of God's children, black men and white men, Jews and Gentiles, Protestants and Catholics, will be able to join hands and sing in the works of the old Negro spiritual: Free at last! Free at last! Thank God Almighty, we are free at last!

Dr. King's words helped our country face the evils of discrimination, and challenged us to work towards building a future founded on a system of social justice and harmony. His words, when joined with actions and deeds, have brought about cooperation and collaboration between people, communities, and institutions in this country and influenced democratic change around the world. Indeed, words can be powerful mechanisms of change.

Another example of the potential power of words is a famous quote from President John F. Kennedy: "Ask not what your country can do for you. Ask what you can do for your country." The late President's remarks invited us to rethink our civic duty in terms of how we could actively contribute to the betterment of our society and its citizenry. His words, like Dr. King's, challenged us to join together and make a commitment to change aimed at improving all humankind. Nichols and Schwartz (1998) noted that John Kennedy's "words had impact because they were carefully chosen and clearly put" (p. 260).

Similarly words, like those used by all helping professionals, have a powerful impact on those hearing the messages. One can well imagine that what is said can be taken to be either positive and empowering, or negative and limiting. In this paper, the authors propose a schema for family-centered practice (Powell, 1996) that supports the need to convey positive empowering messages by framing the helping process around a common egalitarian language and participatory practice approach. Salvador Minuchin (1995) commented that "words like teamwork, co-construction, community, systems, neighborhood, ecology, family, and empowerment began to replace the tired old words like deficit, concern, problems" (p. viii). Thus the schema is offered as a tool for assisting service providers and consumers in making a paradigm shift away from the traditional hierarchically-based helping relationship, where the professional is in charge of the process, to one founded on collaboration between equals.

The core values and principles reflected in the schema are compatible with those found in systems of care. Underpinning the system of care model is a commitment to family focused and child centered service, with the needs of the child and family dictating the type and range of services provided (Stroul & Friedman, 1986). Considered in concert, the system of care represents a conceptual framework for delivering services, and the schema a way in which to make this theoretical design a practice reality.

SYSTEMS OF CARE

The goal of systems of care is to enhance the delivery of mental health services to children and families. To achieve this end, an arrangement for promoting a comprehensive, coordinated range of community-based services has been devised, wherein service providers and consumers work together as equals in the helping process (Powell et al., 1999). In contrast with a continuum of care, a system of care not only includes programs and services, but also embodies a mechanism to ensure that services are provided in a coordinated, cohesive manner. A system of care has been defined as follows:

> A system of care is a comprehensive spectrum of mental health and other necessary services which are organized into a coordinated network to meet the multiple and changing needs of children and adolescents with severe emotional disturbances and their families. (Stroul & Friedman, 1986, p. 3)

Additionally Stroul and Friedman (1996) believe that the core values of a system of care should be: (1) child-centered and family-focused, (2) community-based in terms of services, decision-making, and management responsibility, and (3) culturally sensitive. To actuate the aforementioned values, they suggest the following principles be followed when using the system of care approach: (a) children with emotional disturbances should have access to a comprehensive array of services; (b) children with emotional disturbances should receive services that have been individualized to meet their unique needs; (c) children with emotional disturbances should receive services in the least restrictive, yet clinically appropriate, environment possible; (d) family members should be full participants in all aspects of service planning and delivery of services; (e) children with emotional disturbances should be provided with case management/care coordination to ensure that services are therapeutically appropriate; (f) early identification and early intervention should be promoted; (g) children with emotional disturbances, who reach maturity, should be ensured a smooth transition to the adult service system; (h) advocacy efforts for children with emotional disturbances should be promoted; and (i) services for children with emotional disturbances should be provided with sensitivity and responsiveness to cultural differences and special needs. These values and principles are embedded in the system of care approach, and are central to the helping professional's understanding of and ability to implement the model in practice.

In using the system of care approach, service providers actively engage consumers in the helping process by transferring responsibility for finding therapeutic solutions away from themselves as all-knowing professional experts. Instead, service providers and consumers approach the helping relationship in an equally shared partnership, wherein the responsibility for finding answers and resources is a common goal (Rriesen & Huff, 1996; Koroloff, Friesen, Reilly, & Rinkin, 1996; Osher, defur, Nava, Spencer, & Toth-Dennis, 1999). In this model, families play an active role in need assessment, and service design, delivery, and evaluation. As can be well imagined, full and complete partnership in every aspect of service provision presents challenges for service providers and consumers. Unfortunately, much of the helping language currently in use reinforces the traditional hierarchical therapeutic relationship. The authors believe that the schema's new language can be used to guide helping processes in system of care practice and that its use can help insure that the values and principles of systems of care are enhanced and maintained.

SCHEMA FOR FAMILY-CENTERED PRACTICE

The term schema(s), extracted from the work of Piaget, has been defined by Nichols and Schwartz as "cognitive constructions, or core beliefs, through which people filter their perceptions and structure their experiences" (1998, p. 547). Schemas can therefore provide useful frameworks upon which to organize thoughts and ideas regarding mental health and professional practice. Until the development of the schema for family-centered practice, professional literature contained few user-friendly, family-centered models of practice to guide mental health service providers (Powell, 1996). Unlike the schema, traditional approaches have typically not looked for consumer strengths, but rather focused on deficits thought to exist in the patient or the patient's family. Words and terms like disorder, diagnosis, and treatment, commonly used by exponents of these disease-based practice models, are the antithesis of those used in the schema.

Whereas disease-based terms may be quite useful for physicians and medical personnel treating physical illnesses, they are not compatible with practice concepts founded on a system of care approach. System of care-based practice, according to Fausel (1998), is built upon the following objectives: (1) developing family strengths, (2) helping families become partners with professionals and helping agencies, (3) using a broad range of community and neighborhood resources to help families, and (4) recognizing that each family has a different and unique culture that can be built upon to help families grow stronger.

In particular, the schema is designed to assist service providers and consumers in experiencing the helping process differently from that of traditional pathology driven deficit practice perspectives. It is a less pejorative, more optimistic approach to helping that brings service providers and consumers together in a shared process of growth and discovery. The schema guides service providers and consumers through a cascading series of six steps. The various steps of the schema help organize practice, while at the same time change the basic values upon which the helping process is based. One of the most prominent features of the schema is its terminology, which is shared with and taught to consumers and providers alike.

Learning the skills to become a family-centered practitioner can be confusing for both neophytes and seasoned practitioners. Family-centered practice is not easy; it requires extensive education and supervised experience to develop proficiency. One of the difficulties encountered in developing family-centered skills is the "unlearning" of traditional therapeutic techniques and terminology. Many professionals have been taught terms such as "diagnosis," "treatment," and "termination." Even newer terms like "assessment," "intervention," and "evaluation" are not fully compatible with family-centered practice because they tend to convey professionals as powerful experts (Laird, 1995). Thus, a paradigm shift from traditional to more family-centered, interdisciplinary and collaborative terms is needed. Just as "structural thinking" is more important than technique in structural family therapy (Colapinto, 1983), "system of care thinking" is at the heart of system of care practice.

As a guide to system of care thinking, consider the following steps of the schema:

Joining → Discovery → Change → Celebration → Separation → Reflection

The schema can be thought of as a therapeutic pilgrimage–a journey whereby a family and their child with a serious emotional disturbance, guided by a team of family-centered professionals, can find a more satisfying life. Indeed, the key question that a system of care team should consider when beginning work with a client family is "What does this family need to have a better life?" J. VanDenBerg (personal communication, May 15, 1995).

Practitioners and university students trained with this schema have responded positively. One graduate student said, "It gives me a road map that I have needed and promotes collaboration with families (clients)." Additionally, the six-step schema can be thought of as a rising and spiraling therapeutic process (somewhat like a spiral staircase) whereby families are joined by professional helpers in lifting their lives to more satisfying levels and leading professionals to lifelong quests for excellence in helping.

In general, family therapists and family-centered social workers are moving from directive, hierarchical, and expert stances toward more collaborative coaching relationships with clients (Hartman & Laird, 1983; Nichols & Schwartz, 1998). Also, family-centered practitioners are using family-strengthening, empowering approaches (Berg, 1992; Cole, 1995; de Shazer, 1988; Laird, 1995; Maluccio, 1981; O'Hanlon & Weiner-Davis, 1989; Pinderhughes, 1995; Poulin, 2000; Powell & Dosser, 1992; Saleebey, 1992). Social work literature has long emphasized models of the helping process, but descriptions of process in most models fail to capture the creative, vigorous potential of system of care and family-centered practice.

Each act of helping can build upon a professional's previous experiences, affording a lifelong process of progressive growth in skill and practice wisdom. To return to the image of a spiral staircase, the staircase center post represents the theoretical base that a system of care/ family-centered worker relies upon to anchor his or her practice. Thus the schema can be conceptualized as a spiraling, dynamic process grounded in theory. To help clarify the schema, consider the six steps in more detail:

Joining: Engaging families. Joining is the crucial first step in relationship building. Families seek help for specific problems. They want to learn to cope with life more successfully. Perlman (1989) stated, "The person asking for, or being pushed into, help must be viewed as someone who is trying to cope" (p. 48). To be of help, a system of care team must be able to relate to a family's struggles and at some level be accepted temporarily as a part of a family's system of relationships (Minuchin, 1974).

Families also come into helping relationships with a "history," that is, with their own unique stories. Families need to tell their stories. Families with problems also have many strengths. What successful coping measures have they used in the past?

Discovery: Beyond diagnosis. System of care team members can be conceptualized as "discoverers" who help families explore and nurture their own latent strengths. Discovery advances assessment by emphasizing that families ultimately are the architects and constructors of their own growth and change. System of care workers play important roles as helpers, enablers, and coaches to assist client families to think about and discover their own resources in times of stress.

Discovery replaces such terms a "diagnosis" or "assessment." It implies a collaborative process–not something that is "done to families" but rather a joint client/ team venture. Hartman and Laird (1983) pointed out that social workers could become "coaches" to families while letting families be the principal players. Powell and Dosser (1992) contended that workers could help "too much" by giving advice that robs families of their inherent strengths. During the discovery phase, system of care workers have the opportunity to become "explorers" or "discoverers" with families in a joint exploration of a family's total environment. Such an approach opens possibilities of appreciating the cultural, ethnic, and spiritual uniqueness of a family.

Change: More than treatment. Change implies that family members are the central actors in a helping process. The term change has a positive connotation, implying possibility, even though the change process itself may reflect a time of chaos and instability. Change also suggests a future, hopeful orientation to clients. However, change is a mixture of disequilibrium and growth and can be a difficult process. Colapinto (1982) noted that changing some family systems might require professionals to support individuals within the system while attacking family patterns that limit and restrain growth. Change also assumes that professionals, friends, extended family members and community representatives can and will be willing to examine themselves–asking how they might change their attitudes, policies and practices in order to better assist families.

Celebration: Recognizing and appreciating the strengths and potential in families. Weick and Saleebey (1995) stated, "The legacy of family pathology geared treatment and policy led to even more sophisticated analyses of failure. It has not prepared us to recognize, celebrate, and support family strengths" (p. 147). Celebration does not have to be an ostentatious experience but can be quiet affirmation of growth, potential, confidence, and hope. It is important to celebrate all changes, even subtle ones; if system of care teams and families have a goal of "celebration," something in the course of the helping process that warrants celebrating will likely occur.

Separating: Believing in families' capacity to cope. Dunst and Trivette (1987) noted that empowering families is a process in which " a helper giver takes pride in and derives reward from seeing others become more competent and self-sustaining" (p. 454). Thus workers can take pride in seeing clients leave with greater coping ability.

It is important to help clients "rewrite" their family stories in a more hopeful context. New stories have the potential of changing a family's future, of opening new possibilities and potential for families not only in the present but also in future generations (White, 1992; White & Epston, 1990). Families can carry with them new ways of "coping," with new possibilities, new life, and new meaning open to them. Separation can be a metaphor for setting families free to carry out their life tasks with greater possibilities of success.

Reflection: Opportunity to grow from practice. Reflection can be a post-helping step–a time when families and other system of care team members can think through what has happened. Reflection also implies that family-centered workers have acquired core professional knowledge, skills, and values and that they are constantly adding to their skills and knowledge base through practice wisdom, research (as creators or consumers), continuing education, supervision, and peer consultation. Reflection symbolizes renewal and growth for workers, and each act of helping a family, combined with reflection, has the potential of lifting system of care workers' knowledge, values, and skills to a higher level. Of course, reflection should not occur only at the end of a helping process; it should be a continuous pursuit. Nevertheless, it is important to reflect formally upon an individual or a team's professional work as client families leave the helping relationship. Not only do families learn and grow from professional helpers; helpers also learn and grow from interacting with families. Post-separation reflection can be more than a solitary endeavor; it can involve professional peers as well as family members, with possibilities for group learning and support.

In summary, reflection represents an opportunity for research/evaluation. Workers need to engage in research activities for personal growth as well as to advance that state of family-centered practice. In habitually using the reflection process, professionals and family members develop their skills, as is indicated in the schema by an upward spiral of continuous growth.

FIELD TEST OF THE SCHEMA

The schema was introduced to the staff of the two residential homes for children in Western North Carolina to test its effectiveness in guiding family-centered practice. The authors provided assistance with all aspects of model design, materials, and implementation. Schema materials were distributed to all of the agencies involved in the care of children and families. One of the residential centers specializes in longer-term treatment-oriented placements, and the other shorter, but with a more intense treatment-focused placements. Residential staff from both of the test sites were trained by the authors and selected trainers. The schema was used in a yearlong trial in both agencies. A research process was used to evaluate the schema's effectiveness in: (1) promoting involvement, ownership, voice, and access with families, (2) maintaining focus and intensity with family involvement, (3) increasing satisfaction with the agencies' services, and (4) promoting greater appreciation of the families' own heritage, ethnicity and culture. An analysis of qualitative data confirmed the first three hypotheses, but there were insufficient data to confirm or not confirm the fourth hypothesis (Bass, Dosser & Powell, 2000).

It was clear from reviewing these qualitative data that the schema assisted both workers and families by providing a shared language that promoted partnership. Selected quotes from Bass, Dosser and Powell's (2000) article describing this research demonstrate the utility of the schema and support this conclusion.

Quotes of Staff Members from the Two Agencies

> I am not giving the family the words (any longer). The family has joined in the language and ask questions of each other in new and different ways.

> I often revert to words like "assessment" and "treatment" with the families but it is easy to return to the schema language because they (consumers) have embraced and comfortably use the words of the schema.

> Does it make a difference for the family to have a model? Yes. You want to find tools to get away from using the problem-focused language. The schema matches their vocabulary and fits well with their

vocabulary. The language of the schema does not get in the way of the therapy. It helps the family get away from the pathology language. It helps the family get out of the head and more into the movement and relational part of helping.

With the permission of the family I created a working video tape with the family while utilizing the schema. The tape helped us to realize that the family really familiarized themselves with the language of the schema and felt that the language fit well in their natural environment.

Quotes of Participating Family Members

I think we are discovering now. My stepfather has talked to me more than he ever has. I think the schema helps him.

I keep my schema card in my pocket all the time. It helps me to know where I am and I can check it out with my Dad and see where he thinks we are.

This is my second time here. The schema helps me to understand my folks and how they think. This time I have discovered that I will never be able to go back home to live permanently. The schema has helped me to grow. I will go on to college when I leave here. When I "get crazy" and start getting into trouble I read the back of my schema card and it helps me to settle down and work hard. I will study to be an actor.

She (team-leader) asked us (all of the family members) where we thought we were in the schema model and all of us felt that we were in the process of change. My son felt that he was discovering us for the first time. We all felt that we were in the same place. The schema helped us to know where she felt we were and how many sessions we needed.

SUGGESTIONS FOR USING THE SCHEMA IN SYSTEM OF CARE PRACTICE

The schema is intended as an organizing framework for both providers and consumers of mental health services. It provides them with a language that they can share as well as a common model of the helping process, both of which can increase the sense of partnership and collaboration. As such it is important for both providers and consumers to have easy access to and a clear understanding of the six steps of the schema. Use of training manuals, the schema poster, and schema card have proved useful in this regard. The manual, poster, and card are available from the authors upon request.

Manuals were developed for service providers and consumers. The manuals contained extensive information on the schema including a detailed description of each stage and recommendations for implementing the schema in family-centered practice. Additional commonly used tools (e.g., the genogram, the ecomap, joining strategies, etc.) were described for use in facilitating the work required at each step. These manuals served as the foundation of training for consumers and providers in use of the schema. Although training can vary in terms of content and length, it is imperative that both providers and consumers are trained and share a similar understanding of the schema and its stages. The schema poster and the schema card are also useful in training.

The schema poster (see Figure 1) is an 11-inch by 17-inch poster entitled "Celebrating Change" that presents the schema's six steps in pictorial fashion. High school art students who were provided narrative descriptions of each stage created the pictures representing each stage. The pictures capture the meaning and spirit of each step. For example, discovery is portrayed by a picture of two stick figures (one with a shovel) "discovering" buried treasure. These posters were given to providers and consumers and were prominently displayed in offices and common areas at the residential treatment facilities involved in the research. This facilitated their use during meetings between family members and agency staff. They could easily be referred to as they discussed the schema stages and where they were in the process.

The schema cards are 2 1/4 by 3 3/8-inch laminated cards with the steps of the schema on one side and brief description of each stage on the other side. These cards were developed to provide a quick reference to and summary of the schema. They have been used by providers and consumers and can be easily carried in a wallet or purse. They can be used during meetings with family members and agency staff whether these meetings are formal or informal and whether they are held at the agency, in the family's home, or in another setting. They are most helpful when explaining the schema or its stages to someone.

All of these tools (the training manual, the schema poster, and the schema card) were developed to insure a common frame of reference and a shared understanding of the schema and its implications for family-centered practice. When these tools are available to both consumers and providers of services, it is much more likely that both will share a common language and an understanding of the helping process. This commonality and sharing increase the sense of partnership and collaboration between providers and consumers, which increases the fidelity to the values and principles of system of care thinking and practice.

FIGURE 1

Celebrating Change

A Schema for Family Centered Practice

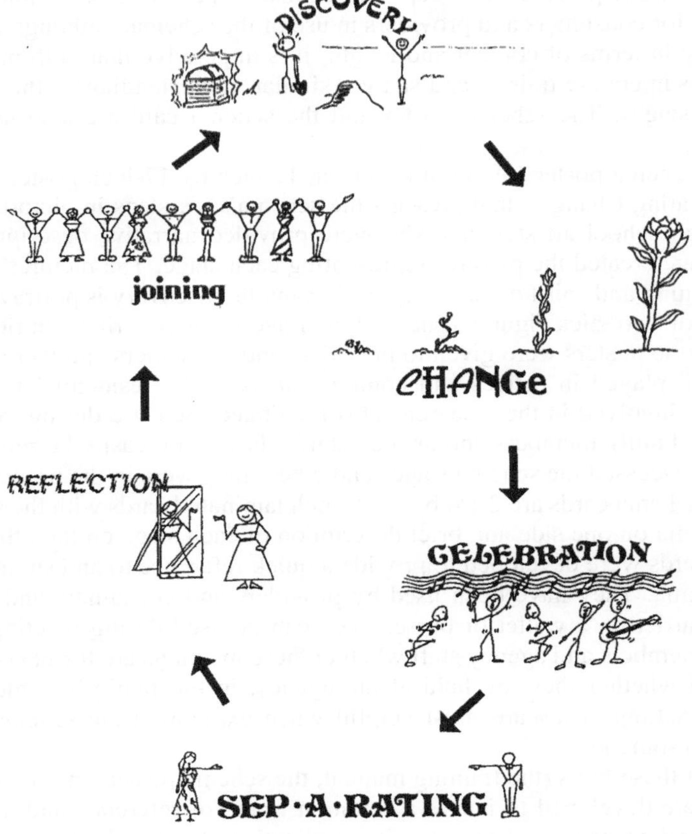

Collaborating to help children and families

REFERENCES

Bass, L.L., Dosser, D.A., Jr., & Powell, J.Y. (2000). Celebrating change: A schema for family-centered practice in residential settings. *Residential Treatment for Children & Youth, 17*(3), 123-137.

Berg, I.K. (1992). *Family-based service: A solution focused approach.* Milwaukee, WI: Brief Family Therapy Center.

Colapinto, J. (1982). Structural family therapy. In A.M. Horne & M.M. Ohlsen (Eds.), *Family Counseling and Therapy* (pp. 112-140). Itasca, IL: F.E. Peacock.

Colapinto, J. (1983). Beyond technique: Teaching how to think structurally. *Journal of Strategic and Systemic Therapies, 2*(2), 12-21.

Cole, E.S. (1995). Becoming family-centered: Child welfare's challenge. *Families in Society, 76,* 163-172.

De Shazer, S. (1988). *Clues: Investigating solutions in brief therapy.* New York: W.W. Norton.

Dunst, C.J., Trivette, C.M. (1987). Enabling and empowering families: Conceptual and intervention issues. *School Psychology Review, 16,* 443-456.

Fausel, D. F. (1998). Collaborative conversations for change: A solution focused approach to family-centered practice. *Family Preservation Journal, 3*(1), 59-74.

Friesen, B.J., & Huff, B. (1996). Family perspectives on systems of care. In. B.A. Stroul (Ed.), *Children's Mental Health: Creating Systems of Care in a Changing Society* (pp.41-67). Baltimore, MD: Brookes.

Hartman, A., & Laird, J. (1983). *Family-centered social work practice.* New York: Free Press.

Koroloff, N.M. & Friesen, B.J., Reilly, L., Rinkin, J. (1996). The role of family members in systems of care. In B.A. Stroul (Ed.), *Children's Mental Health; Creating Systems of Care in a Changing Society* (pp. 409-426). Baltimore, MD: Brookes.

Laird, J. (1995). Family-centered practice in the postmodern era. *Families in Society, 76,* 150-162.

Maluccio, A.N. (1981). *Promoting competence in clients: A new/old approach to social work practice.* New York: Free Press.

Minuchin, S. (1974). *Families and family therapy.* Cambridge, MA: Harvard University Press.

Minuchin, S. (1995). A simple fable for a complex problem (foreword). In P. Adams & K. Nelson (Eds.), *Reinventing Human Services: Community-and-family-centered practice.* New York: Aldire DeGruyter.

Nichols, M.P., & Schwartz, R.C. (1998). *Family therapy: Concepts and methods* (4th ed.). Boston, MA: Allyn & Bacon.

O'Hanlon, B., & Weiner-Davis, M. (1989). *In search of solutions: A new direction in psychotherapy.* New York: W.W. Norton.

Osher, T.W., de Fur, E., Nava, C., Spencer, S., & Toth-Dennis, D. (1999). New roles for families in systems of care. In *Systems of Care: Promising Practices in Children's Mental Health 1998 Series, Volume 1.* Washington, DC: Center for Effective Collaboration and Practice, American Institutes for Research.

Perlman, H.H. (1989). *Looking back to see ahead.* Chicago: University of Chicago Press.

Pinderhughes, E. (1995). Empowering divers populations: Family practice in the 21st century. *Families in Society, 76*, 131-140.

Poulin, J. (2000). *Collaborative social work: Strengths-based generalist practice.* Itaska, IL: F. E. Peacock.

Powell, J.Y. (1996). A schema for family-centered practice. *Families in Society, 77*(7), 446-448.

Powell, J., Dosser, D., Handron, D., McCammon, S.,Temkin, M. E., Kaufman, M. (1999). Challenges of interdisciplinary collaboration: A faculty consortiums initial attempts to model collaborative practice. *Journal of Community Practice, 6*(2), 27-48.

Powell, J.Y., & Dosser, D.A. (1992). Structural family therapy as a bridge between "helping too much" and empowerment. *Family Therapy, 19*, 243-256.

Saleebey, D. (Ed.). (1992). *The strengths perspective in social work practice.* New York: Longman.

Stroul, B. & Friedman, R. (1986). *A system of care for children and youth with severe emotional disturbances* (Rev. ed.). Washington, DC: Georgetown University Child Development Center, National Technical Assistance Center for Children's Mental Health.

Stroul, B. & Friedman, R. (1996). The system of care concept and philosophy. In B. A. Stroul (Ed.), *Children's Mental Health: Creating Systems of Care in a Changing Society* (pp. 3-21). Baltimore, MD: Paul. H. Brookes.

Weick, A., & Saleebey, D. (1995). Supporting family strengths: Orienting policy and practice toward the 21st century. *Families in Society, 76*, 141-149.

White, M. (1992, October 17). *Recent developments in the narrative approach.* Paper presented at the American Association of Marriage and Family Therapy, Miami, FL.

White, M., & Epston, D. (1990). *Narrative means to a therapeutic ends.* New York: W.W. Norton.

Challenges of Providing Interdisciplinary Mental Health Education

Dorothea Handron, EdD
John Diamond, MD
Joan Levy Zlotnik, PhD, ACSW

SUMMARY. Recommendations and implications of the Pew Health Professions Commission's fourth and final report emphasized the importance of developing interdisciplinary competencies for health professionals (Bellack & O'Neil, 2000). Headrick and Moore (1999) reported to the Association of Academic Health Centers that interprofessional collaboration has not been easy, in part, because most health professional faculty are products of individual, discipline specific models for education. This article provides a conceptual foundation for interdisci-

---

Dorothea Handron is Associate Professor, Department of Community Nursing Services, School of Nursing and John Diamond is Director and Associate Professor, Department of Psychiatry, Division of Child and Adolescent Psychiatry, Brody School of Medicine, East Carolina University. Joan Levy Zlotnik is Executive Director, Institute for the Advancement of Social Work Research, Washington, DC.

Address correspondence to: Dorothea Handron, School of Nursing, Rivers Building, East Carolina University, Greenville, NC 27858-4353 (E-mail: handrond@mail.ecu.edu).

Appreciation is expressed to Ms. Traci Lynch for assistance in manuscript preparation.

Preparation of the manuscript was funded in part through a contract with the North Carolina Division of Mental Health, Developmental Disabilities and Substance Abuse Services, Child and Family Services, as a component of the System of Care: Training and Curriculum Development Project, funded by a grant from the Center for Mental Health Services.

[Haworth co-indexing entry note]: "Challenges of Providing Interdisciplinary Mental Health Education." Handron, Dorothea, John Diamond, and Joan Levy Zlotnik. Co-published simultaneously in *Journal of Family Social Work* (The Haworth Social Work Practice Press, an imprint of The Haworth Press, Inc.) Vol. 5, No. 3, 2001, pp. 49-62; and: *Child Mental Health: Exploring Systems of Care in the New Millennium* (ed: David A. Dosser, Jr. et al.) The Haworth Social Work Practice Press, an imprint of The Haworth Press, Inc., 2001, pp. 49-62. Single or multiple copies of this article are available for a fee from The Haworth Document Delivery Service [1-800-342-9678, 9:00 a.m. - 5:00 p.m. (EST). E-mail address: getinfo@haworthpressinc.com].

© 2001 by The Haworth Press, Inc. All rights reserved.

plinary health care education at the graduate level based on findings from an interdisciplinary course in child/family mental health at East Carolina University. Classroom challenges affecting interdisciplinary offerings and specific problems that preclude integration of medical students are addressed. The article offers strategies to create a positive interdisciplinary learning climate for pre-professional education. Evidenced-based medicine is discussed as a mechanism to remove discipline specific barriers. *[Article copies available for a fee from The Haworth Document Delivery Service: 1-800-342-9678. E-mail address: <getinfo@haworthpressinc.com> Website: <http://www.HaworthPress.com> © 2001 by The Haworth Press, Inc. All rights reserved.]*

KEYWORDS. Interdisciplinary education, collaborative practice, teaching methods, classroom barriers, evidence-based practice

Recommendations and implications of the Pew Health Professions Commission's fourth and final report issued in December of 1998 assessed the challenges facing health care professionals in the 21st century. These general and profession-specific recommendations strongly emphasized the importance of developing interdisciplinary competencies for health professionals.

Recognizing that interdisciplinary competence has not been a priority in health professions education, the Commission urged schools in the health professions to provide 25% or more of their clinical education in settings that model or support interdisciplinary practice (Bellack & O'Neil, 2000). The report suggested that students be provided learning opportunities in interdisciplinary teamwork possibly using case-based or problem-based learning experiences that demonstrate how various health profession disciplines can work together. It provided a strong mandate for educators in the health professions to change current structures and policies that limit opportunities for interdisciplinary teaching or learning, in order to meet the demands of the new health care system (Bellack & O'Neal, 2000).

Headrick and Moore (1999) reported to the Association of Academic Health Centers that interprofessional collaborations have not been easy or natural for health care professionals. Most professionals are trained in individual problem solving and decision-making rather than using collaborative team approaches to service delivery. Because of the complexity of health care issues and systems, multiple perspectives must now be "brought to bear on many health problems" (p. 1). The issue is further complicated in that most health professional faculty are products of individual, discipline specific models for education. They are, therefore, ill equipped to use or teach interdisciplinary education approaches.

Interdisciplinary course offerings challenge higher education to move rapidly into a "brave new world." What happens in the interdisciplinary classroom, when students from various health care or social science disciplines work together, often blurring the lines between discipline specific areas of expertise, to develop inclusive, collaborative plans for patients, families and children with serious physical or emotional needs? These classes are usually facilitated by a plurality of faculty representing students' disciplines, and parent/patient advocates who forthrightly articulate their problems with existing service delivery. These key "players" contribute to creating a complex, highly charged learning environment that has not been carefully studied.

Several factors emerge as challenges to fostering interdisciplinary collaborative education in university settings. Within the classroom, competitive behaviors of students and faculty put a damper on interdisciplinary processes. Larger system constraints between departments in universities affect the ability to schedule such courses and include a broad range of interdisciplinary participants. The expense of having multiple faculty cover one course and fair distribution of faculty workload in interdisciplinary teaching are significant obstacles to overcome. Finally, medical school curricula, schedules and biases keep medical students, and physicians who train them, from taking part in interdisciplinary health education activities.

This article provides a theoretical and conceptual foundation for interdisciplinary education. It defines the classroom challenges that may occur when implementing this type of graduate level course based on findings from a course at East Carolina University. Strategies are included to establish a learning climate for an ecological approach to interdisciplinary practice in pre-professional education that encourages medical student participation.

CONCEPTUAL FRAMEWORK FOR INTERDISCIPLINARY EDUCATION

Professional literature is rampant with statements supporting the importance of collaborative practice. It is generally agreed that health care consumers, families, professionals, educators, spiritual leaders and community members should be, and in many instances, are already being invited to work together to address complex needs for children, families, and all health care service users. Collaboration, the watchword for these interactions, is defined "as a process to reach goals that cannot be achieved acting singly" (Bruner, as cited in Osher, defur, Nava, Spencer, & Toth-Dennis, 1999, p. 3). Davis, Litrownik, and Weinstein (1997), in describing an interdisciplinary education initiative related to child abuse and neglect, suggested that collaboration to arrive at agreed upon case goals requires the acquisition of cross-disciplinary knowledge as well as the development of an interdisciplinary attitude and skills in interdisciplinary communication and collaboration. Collaboration involves shared responsibility, shared goals and working together (Osher et al., 1999). Another approach is taken by Houle, Cyphert, and Boggs (1987), who defined interprofessional education as the communication, cooperation and coordination that occurs between members of two or more professions when they are dealing with client concerns that extend beyond the usual area of any one profession. In order for collaborative dialogue to take place, Seaburn Lorenz, Gunn, Gawinski and Mauksch (1998) suggested the importance of three basic tenets (1) an integrative paradigm exists to respond to health and mental health difficulties; (2) an ecological perspective is used as a basis for interactions between collaborating professionals and; (3) health care consumers, clients and families are partners in care.

An integrative paradigm provides a holistic framework for considering the strengths and needs of a child, family or service user. In the past, professional disciplines tended to adapt reductionistic, deficit-based, bio/psycho/social models when offering consultation to clients. A specific discipline's theoretical view of clients' concerns often related to "pre-packaged interventions" or categorical services that were readily available. For example, physicians relied on a biological model amenable to treatment by medications, which they prescribed. Nurses were influenced by bio/psycho/social factors because their interventions included therapeutic communication and altering environmental factors. The realms of social work and psychology have been psychosocial and emphasized behavioral phenomena that existed outside the purview of the medical model. Family therapists claimed the usefulness of family systems and structural theories, and based their interventions accordingly. For all, these "guild" interventions were primarily discipline based, not evidence based.

An integrative paradigm encompasses physical, emotional, social, cultural and spiritual factors that influence the health and well-being of children, individuals, families and communities (Amara et al., 1998). Within this paradigm, a problem or need of a client or family is explored within a broader, inclusive context where helping resources may be more readily available. Professional and client/family teams focus on needs as determined by the service user, and by an increasing emphasis on intervention plans that are evidence based.

An ecological approach suggests that professionals, service users, and families focus on the process of interactions between them in order to maintain a broad, realistic perception of clients' needs and the availability of shared resources. This approach supports transdisciplinary health care teams oriented towards the process of care and outcomes that actively incorporate the patient's family into the treatment process. The team continuously monitors progress from the perspectives of each discipline, but with the ultimate goal of formulating a completely integrated approach (Firpo, 1999).

The process of communication within teams using an ecological approach is equal in importance to content that is being discussed (Seaburn et al.,

1998). It does not mandate that professionals from different disciplines abandon their theoretical perspectives in favor of emphasizing communications techniques. Inherent to this approach however, is the belief that all participants relinquish the supremacy of their theoretical frameworks of origin when working in collaboration (Seaburn et al., 1998). Herein lies the challenge for many professionals who engage in collaborative efforts without the knowledge or skills to use a holistic, process oriented, and evidence-based ecological approach. Proponents of an ecological approach maintain that the quality of inclusive, open communication is a significant predictor for successful treatment outcomes for complex problems. How do we adequately prepare professionals during pre-professional education to actively engage in this kind of dialogue and potentiate interdisciplinary team practice?

Collaborative practice techniques are especially relevant for professionals working in child and family mental health (Powell et al., 1999; Stroul, 1996). During team meetings, stereotypical attitudes towards health care consumers and families are often covertly manifested. These attitudes imply that health care consumers and families are, at the very least, dependent on the expertise of professionals, and at most, don't understand the root of their own problems. Professional education in mental health disciplines gives lip service to changing these attitudes among their own ranks. To realistically initiate changes in these deeply ingrained beliefs, family members and health care consumers must be included as equal partners in university classrooms as teachers and facilitators for pre-professional training.

Collaborative practice is the umbrella for interdisciplinary, multidisciplinary and transdisciplinary approaches being used throughout the nation. Many pre-professional mental health care, behavioral and social science disciplines now include interdisciplinary components (Holmes & Osterweis, 1999). These students share clinical sites and work in teams caring for clients and families. They attend interdisciplinary team meetings in agencies and form interesting opinions about the work scope and biases of their peers in other disciplines. Often, in an attempt to foster positive working relationships, several disciplines on a university campus attend symposia or workshops to share information. Innovative on-line courses and university partnerships bring various disciplines together in shared content areas. Courses on interdisciplinary practice, such as those at Case Western Reserve University and at the University of Texas at Houston, are beginning to be offered at universities throughout the nation (Headrick & Moore, 1999; Holmes & Osterweis, 1999). What these endeavors share is providing students the opportunity to understand the knowledge, value and ethical base of other professions, which should assist them in learning to work together. Interdisciplinary education can usually be identified by 3 components: (1) coursework related to team work and collaboration; (2) different disciplines studying shared content together, e.g., child development or child abuse; and (3) shared field work or internship opportunities.

However, most of these interdisciplinary courses have not been mainstreamed into graduate core curriculums or university cultures. They remain elective offerings that only a few students choose to take. They are often scheduled during less populated summer sessions and require external funding. Generally, interdisciplinary practice courses do not include medical students, though physicians are often members of mental health practice teams.

INTERDISCIPLINARY EDUCATION: CHALLENGES AFFECTING STUDENTS AND FACULTY

A campus based, cross listed course on interdisciplinary practice was developed at East Carolina University (ECU), a result of a community partnership between ECU and mental health agencies in three rural eastern North Carolina counties serving children and families with serious emotional disorders. What makes this course unique, from several others offered, is that it focuses on how to engage in interdisciplinary practice as opposed to studying professional issues from interdisciplinary or multidisciplinary perspectives. It has been offered the past four years to students in Departments of Psychology and Child and Family Relations and the Schools of Social Work and Nursing.

Student and faculty responses to participation in these classes have been carefully evaluated and offer significant insights into the challenges associated with interdisciplinary education. Participating graduate students are from various health professions and social science disciplines, and they vary widely in age, prior life experiences, professional expectations, maturity, and attitudes. In an unpublished paper by Handron (1998), graduate students at ECU taking these classes on interdisciplinary practice, expressed a variety of concerns. Foremost they felt threatened in a classroom with students and faculty from other disciplines, sensing "professional outsiders" were judging them more critically. To safeguard feeling vulnerable, these students closely monitored or limited their contributions during class discussions. Role-play activities to develop communication skills for interdisciplinary team practice were particularly anxiety provoking for many who felt they were "on stage performing in front of other disciplines." Practicing conflict resolution skills, a significant component of any interdisciplinary learning experience, was particularly problematic for students attempting to suppress their own insecurities and conflictual feelings about classmates and faculty from other disciplines. If these "isolationist" dynamics remain unchallenged, then participation and learning in an interdisciplinary class is likely to be seriously compromised.

Furthermore, many interesting "turf" issues emerged in these interdisciplinary classes. Conflicts arose from students' uninformed or unrealistic rationales for making their career choices. By the time these students entered an interdisciplinary class (usually at senior undergraduate or graduate levels), they had developed strong alliances to their adopted professional cultures. They were knowledgeable about the tasks and expertise that were included within the boundaries of their disciplines, and they believed they had a good sense about what other disciplines were supposed to do in practice. Imagine their surprise when they discovered that in the current health care arena, boundaries for professional practice are blurred and skewed. More than one discipline may engage in similar professional activities and claim expertise in areas that overlap. This also affects the notion of compensation in a world where health care dollars and resources are already seriously limited. Who will likely be hired, the psychiatrist, or the advanced practice nurse who may offer similar services? Questions of this nature prompted many students to feel insecure about their professional choices. Though these tensions may be normal, they must be normalized and "revisited" often in an interdisciplinary class.

Faculty members shared many of the same concerns as students when they participated in interdisciplinary classes. "How will I be judged by my colleagues from other disciplines?" Traditional rivalries between disciplines surfaced with faculty members co-teaching the interdisciplinary course at ECU. For example, physicians and nurses were particularly challenged to avoid acting out stereotypes regarding traditional professional leadership patterns. Disciplines have unique academic cultures, rigor regarding educational content and licensing, and various time perspectives, which can affect their teaching styles and evaluation methods. It is easy to devalue a colleague's approach to teaching based on a different professional style. Academicians earn their salaries by sharing knowledge with others through spoken and written words. With more than one discipline "sharing the floor" in an interdisciplinary classroom, it is likely that all faculty participants will feel obligated to offer an opinion. This provides for a lively dialogue between faculty and often leaves students sitting quietly, feeling overwhelmed and being un-involved in a discussion.

Barriers for student and faculty participation in interdisciplinary education can be successfully countered. Strong group facilitation and processing skills are integral to the success of any interdisciplinary educational experience. Awareness concerning the heightened sensitivities of students regarding "performing" in front of other disciplines should be taken into account when developing practice type role-play exercises. Faculty must closely monitor class discussions in which heated exchanges serve to immobilize students rather than stimulate their thinking.

Time is well spent in any interdisciplinary class that focuses on discipline specific assumptions and cultural stereotypes. Handron (1998) described an assignment in which students in an interdisciplinary class were required to study another discipline by visiting their classes, and interviewing students and faculty in other departmental settings. Class presentations reflected that this learning exercise successfully challenged negative stereotypes and biases about other professionals. Realistic perceptions about other professional cultures naturally emerged and were validated by class participants from those disciplines who were taking the interdisciplinary class. Students were encouraged to discuss their concerns and frustrations about interdisciplinary practice and usually discovered that they shared common insecurities and practice issues. This awareness altered their sense of being threatened by others, and it provoked an open exchange of ideas.

To insure the success of an interdisciplinary offering, faculty must be highly invested in being participants. This is particularly important because few other professional rewards exist at this time in academia for faculty involved in innovative interdisciplinary teaching (Fulginiti, 1999). Because this type of collaborative teaching can be threatening, even for the seasoned professional, relationship building between faculty participants should be a primary undertaking prior to preparing an interdisciplinary class. Faculty will value opportunities to get to know each other in non-threatening environments. Here, they are encouraged to share their notions on teaching, professional interests, and the strengths they bring both to the classroom and clinical practice. As part of the relationship building, they can engage in personal socialization. Teaching teams, who take the time to get to know each other, and develop a sense of trust and mutual respect, will be most effective in role modeling positive working relationships for their students. The faculty will then be prepared for such events as when students "unintentionally" pit them against each other regarding assignments; these problems can be dealt with forthrightly and positively in a manner that prompts many positive interdisciplinary insights.

It is difficult to find experienced mentors trained in the model (Brandon and Meuter, 1995). Fulginiti (1999) emphasized the need for faculty to be trained in interdisciplinary teaching. Faculty discipline cultures that rely on lecture formats will be particularly challenged by interdisciplinary education. These types of offerings are most effective when small group experiential instructional methods are used.

Sites (1997) suggested that it is helpful to have a neutral place to foster interdisciplinary efforts in the university such as in the Vice President's or Provost's Office. The University of Pittsburgh has an Office of Child Development, in the provost's office that develops grants and also coordinates interdisciplinary child welfare efforts, decreasing conflict and competition among different disciplines. A center for professional interdisciplinary education, as established in the Health Sciences Division at East Carolina University, is helpful in providing specialized teaching resources, staff development, cross professional interactions, and incentives for university faculty (Holmes & Osterweis, 1999).

Teaching methods that are appropriate for interdisciplinary teaching might include:

- Case study
- Real-life community problem-solving design
- Participation in field work, site-based interdisciplinary teams and seminars in teams
- Team teaching
- Student support seminars
- Field instructors becoming adjunct faculty
- Interactive learning among faculty, students and the community
- Families/parents/consumers teaching in the classroom (Brandon & Meuter, 1996)

It is helpful to establish a faculty point person with one assistant when multiple interdisciplinary faculty are involved in classroom teaching. Though all faculty should determine class content, a form of tag teaching in which no more than two specific faculty assume responsibility for teaching an individual class, limits faculty interactions and insures greater student participation.

Interdisciplinary teaching is *not* time efficient for faculty. It requires considerable time for group pre-planning and evaluation. When planning and meeting times are configured, interdisciplinary teaching time requires double that of a single course.

Faculty participants may divide grading of assignments between themselves though all should be involved in creating the evaluation measures. When one assignment is graded entirely by a specific faculty member, students' concerns about consistent grading on that assignment are eliminated. Group presentations are an important and worthwhile evaluation tool in any interdisciplinary education endeavor. Faculty and other teaching resources (parent advocates) should participate in providing positive feedback about these presentations. This unique opportunity for students to gain insights about their work from a variety of sources may be what is best about interdisciplinary education.

BARRIERS TO INTERDISCIPLINARY EDUCATION WITH THE MEDICAL CAMPUS

Medical education in mental health often begins during the first year of medical school and is usually the domain of departments of psychiatry. The curriculum includes normal psychological development and the study of psychopathology. This is the first opportunity for interdisciplinary education, which is often missed. It is dependent on who is assigned to teach the course, and the resources available to the department. If the department of psychiatry functions as an interdisciplinary unit, then this model is often presented to the medical students. As departments of psychiatry consolidate with rising financial pressures from managed care, they are becoming, more and more, physician only departments. This may be promoted by deans and chairs who emphasize the apprenticeship guild model, implying that only physicians can teach physicians.

Basic behavioral science courses are followed by a clinical experience in psychiatry, typically in the third year of medical school. The medical model is strongest in the hospital setting, and students are usually placed on inpatient psychiatric units. Treatment on these units has traditionally relied on the milieu, which provides an opportunity for disciplines to draw upon their unique strengths in the service of patients. From psychiatry, social work and psychology to recreation therapy, occupational therapy and nursing, each discipline contributes its own assessment style and theoretical framework to patient care. In this setting, interdisciplinary education for medical students is dependent on the orientation and personality of the medical director. At best, students can learn the clinical role of each discipline. But they are not exposed to an integrative model allowing disciplines to complement each other. In some ways, managed care has led to a retrenchment from this model. Average lengths of stay are now too short for a true milieu approach, staff numbers have been reduced, and stabilization is often left to pharmacological interventions. Although the biopsychosocial model is the buzzword, the biological aspect reigns supreme.

Medical students have other opportunities for interdisciplinary education during clinical rotations. On medical units, they may find an enlightened attending physician who has more interest in psychosocial aspects of illness. Particularly when exposed to chronic or terminal illnesses, there may be teams composed of nurses, psychologists and social workers. The advent of family medicine as a specialty, replacing the non-specialized general practitioner, has led to an even greater use of multidisciplinary teams. Family Medicine programs were among the first to incorporate pharmacists and dieticians along with nurses, psychologists and social workers in treating families more holistically. Even with these progressive initiatives, academic medical settings have not advanced to using integrative models. The physician is maintained as team leader. One of the reasons cited are legal concerns about "ultimate" responsibility. Medical malpractice remains a reality issue, which maintains physician dominance. Although clinical responsibility may be shared, the courts have not relieved physicians of ultimate legal responsibilities. Another factor is the vague notion of clinical experience. Although the concept of clinical experience has been shown to often represent invalid evidence and poor decision-making (Sackett, 1998), it has remained an excuse, even in the face of competing evidence, for physicians to have the final word in team meetings.

Various structural barriers also preclude medical students' participation in interdisciplinary classes. Medical education is unlike other forms of graduate education. Students are in class daily, often for eight hours. There are no electives until late in the curriculum, and those are not based on the semester system. Graduation is not based on credit hours or a thesis, but on successful completion of a rigorous academic curriculum. This has historically prevented classroom cross training with other graduate disciplines oriented towards credit hours and semesters. Time constraints for inclusion of mandatory medical curriculum content preclude opportunities for students to participate in elective interdisciplinary courses. Additional challenges are related to the difficulty in scheduling shared field education experiences due to the diverse schedules of different disciplines (Knapp et al., 1994), and concerns regarding meeting licensing or other credentialing requirements in specific disciplines (Hogan, 1996; Lawson, 1996).

As mental health disciplines attempt to work together within the medical realm, their lack of shared classroom experiences prevents developing a common theoretical basis for practice. More enlightened programs may cross-teach, where a psychiatrist could teach a course on psychopharmacology to graduate social work students, or a marriage and family therapist may teach a course on therapy to psychiatry residents. But these exceptions are uncommon, and the amount of time for cross-discipline exposure is insufficient for gaining much more than an appreciation of each other's existence. Patients and families serving as teachers or consultants rarely enter the university classroom of medical students.

These structural barriers and limited exposure to professionals outside the medical guild preclude the development of novel interdisciplinary coursework and clinical experiences. Biases about other disciplines or service users are transmitted and are slowly etched into the minds of medical students. Unfortunately, these early biases and barriers are maintained between physicians and other disciplines long after they enter the world of practice.

An integrative paradigm change in the educational model, serving to break the guild barrier, could be evidence-based medicine. The Evidence Based Medicine movement (EBM) values the objective demonstration of treatment efficacy in double blind, randomized, controlled clinical trials above clinical experience, local experts, and other sources where potential biases have not been identified or controlled.

The use of EBM techniques in an interdisciplinary class has the potential to remove discipline barriers and support physician training. In this model, decisions are made not by clinical experience or administrative fiat, but rather by the best evidence supporting a positive outcome. For example, the following case study of a team meeting at a residential treatment center, with a clinically depressed adolescent might be used in an interdisciplinary class. The physician wants to prescribe an antidepressant. The psychologist is interested in cognitive-behavioral therapy, while the social worker thinks there are problems in the parental subsystem and wants to utilize structural family therapy. The parent is confused, and maybe even biased by whatever approach their case manager is advocating. A traditional approach may well lead to the physician making the final determination that medication is most clearly indicated, perhaps citing personal "experience with these kinds of cases." An astute nurse presents a Med-Line search that fails to demonstrate evidence for efficacy of antidepressants in adolescents. The search finds the most compelling evidence for cognitive-behavioral therapy. The final decision is not based on the winning perspective of one discipline, but by evidence from the vast multidisciplinary literature.

CONCLUSION

Fulginiti (1999) concludes that interdisciplinary professional education is "the right thing to do at the right time in the history of academe, education, research, and clinical care." However educators must "approach this activity as rigorously as we do the other parts of our academic effort" (1999, p. 22). Unfortunately, the creation and establishment of new interdisciplinary education programs are assumed to be either: (1) Fraught with barriers that probably can't be overcome, or (2) Incredibly easy to teach–JUST DO IT! Neither of these beliefs are true.

Greenberg and Bellack (1999) offer the following suggestions to foster interdisciplinary education and practice culture. First, define and conceptualize what interdisciplinary practice means, and communicate it throughout the institution. Interdisciplinary learning experiences should be required within curricula rather than being elective, and this content should be introduced early to students pursuing health or social science disciplines. Capitalize on students' natural interest and enthusiasm for working together and learning from each other before they become entrenched in their individual professional guilds. Create faculty incentives to engage in interdisciplinary teaching and build these into promotion, tenure and merit award criteria.

Finally, physicians in training must be included in interdisciplinary courses. An effective means of bringing physicians into interdisciplinary training may be through emphasizing evidence-based practice content. Perhaps the most evidence-based aspect of the entire interdisciplinary teaching effort would be our ability to demonstrate improved outcomes for children and families due to interdisciplinary education and training.

REFERENCES

Amara, R., Cain, M., Cypress, D., Dempsey, H., Everett, W., Falcon, R., Holt, M., Kyrouz, E., Mittmand, R., Morrison, I., Pascali, M., Schmid, G., Wilson, C., & Yu, K. (1998). *A Forecast of Health and Health Care in America: The Future Beyond 2005* (Institute for the future). Princeton, NJ: The Robert Wood Johnson Foundation.

Bellack, J. P. & O'Neil, E. H. (2000). Recreating nursing practice for a new century. *Nursing and Health Care Perspectives, 21*(1), 14-21.

Brandon, R., & Meuter, L. (1995). Proceedings of the National Conference on Interprofessional Education and Training, Los Angeles, CA, March 23-25, 1995. Seattle, WA: Human Services Policy Center, University of Washington.

Davis, I., Litrownik, A., & Weinstein, J. (1997). Levels of interdisciplinary education for child welfare practice: A report of the San Diego Interdisciplinary child welfare training (ICWT) Project, San Diego State University, School of Social Work.

Firpo, A. (1999). Tools for effective leadership in the 21st Century. In D. E. Holmes & M. Osterweis (Eds.), *Catalysts in Interdisciplinary Education* (pp. 117-136). Washington, DC: Association of Academic Health Centers.

Fulginiti, V. A., (1999). The right issue at the right time. In D. E. Holmes, & M. Osterweis (Eds.), *Catalysts in Interdisciplinary Education* (pp. 7-25). Washington, DC: Association of Academic Health Centers.

Greenberg, R. S., & Bellack, J. P. (1999). Building an interdisciplinary culture. In D. E. Holmes, & M. Osterweis (Eds.), *Catalysts in Interdisciplinary Education* (pp. 59-79). Washington, DC: Association of Academic Health Centers.

Handron, D. (1998). A pilot study of interdisciplinary practice course: Learning as we move forward. Paper presented at Vice Chancellor's Symposium for Interdisciplinary Education. East Carolina University, Greenville, North Carolina.

Headrick, L. A., & Moore, S. M., (1999). *Factors in the success of one faculty team's experience in interprofessional education.* Washington, DC: Association of Academic Health Centers.

Hogan, P. (1996). Transforming professional education. In K. Hooper-Briar & H. Lawson (Eds.), *Expanding partnerships for vulnerable children, youth and families*, (pp. 222-230). Alexandria, VA: CSWE.

Holmes, D. E., & Osterweis, M. (Eds.) (1999). *Catalysts in Interdisciplinary Education.* Washington, DC: Association of Academic Health Centers.

Houle, C., Cyphert, F. & Boggs, D. (Spring, 1987). Education for the professions. *Theory into practice: Interprofessional education, 26*(2).

Knapp, M., Barnard, K, Brandon, R., Gehrke, N., Smith, A. & Teather, E. (1994). University-based preparation for collaborative interprofessional practice. In L. Adler & S. Gardner (Eds.), *The politics of linking schools and social services*, (pp. 137-152). Washington, DC: Falmer Press.

Lawson, H. (1996). Credentialing issues for interprofessional education and practice. In K. Hooper-Briar & H. Lawson (Eds.), *Expanding partnerships for vulnerable children, youth and families* (pp. 203-221). Alexandria, VA: CSWE.

Osher, T. W., Defur, E., Nava, C., Spencer, S., & Toth-Dennis, D. (1999). New roles for families in systems of care. In *Systems of Care Promising Practices in Chil-*

dren's Mental Health 1998 Series, 1. Washington, DC: Center for Effective Collaboration and Practice, American Institutes for Research.

Powell, J., Dosser, D., Handron, D., McCammon, S., Temkin, M. E., & Kaufman, M. (1999). Challenges of interdisciplinary collaboration: A faculty consortium's initial attempts to model collaborative practice. *Journal of Community Practice, 6*(2), 27-47.

Sackett, D. L., Richardson, W. S., Rosenberg W., & Haynes, R. B. (1998). *Evidence-based Medicine: How to Practice and Teach EBM.* New York: Churchill Livingstone.

Seaburn, D. B., Lorenz, A. D., Gunn, W. B. Jr., Gawinski, B. A. & Mauksch, L. B. (1996). *Models of Collaboration.* New York: Basic Books.

Sites, E. (1997). Final Report to the Children's Bureau of the University of Pittsburgh, Child Welfare Interdisciplinary Training Grant, University of Pittsburgh, School of Social Work.

Stroul, B. (1996). *Children's Mental Health: Creating systems of care in a changing society.* Baltimore, MD: Paul H. Brookes.

Including Families' Spiritual Beliefs and Their Faith Communities in Systems of Care

David A. Dosser, Jr., PhD
Angela L. Smith, PhD
Edward W. Markowski, PhD
Harry I. Cain, MA

SUMMARY. System of care (SOC) philosophy and principles were developed and systems of care are designed and implemented to improve the mental health services that are delivered to children and families. The identification and effective use of resources to assist

David A. Dosser, Jr. is Director and Associate Professor, Angela L. Smith is Assistant Professor, Edward W. Markowski is Professor, and Harry I. Cain is Adjunct Faculty member, Marriage and Family Therapy Program, Department of Child Development and Family Relations, School of Human Environmental Sciences, East Carolina University.

Address correspondence to: David A. Dosser, Marriage and Family Therapy Program, Rivers Building, East Carolina University, Greenville, NC 27858-4353 (E-mail: dosserd@mail.ecu.edu).

Appreciation is expressed to Ms. Traci Lynch for assistance in manuscript preparation.

Preparation of the manuscript was funded in part through a contract with the North Carolina Division of Mental Health, Developmental Disabilities and Substance Abuse Services, Child and Family Services, as a component of the System of Care: Training and Curriculum Development Project, funded by a grant from the Center for Mental Health Services.

Portions of this paper were presented at the Annual Conference of the North Carolina Association for Marriage and Family Therapy on March 12, 1999 in Greensboro, NC.

[Haworth co-indexing entry note]: "Including Families' Spiritual Beliefs and Their Faith Communities in Systems of Care." Dosser, David A., Jr. et al. Co-published simultaneously in *Journal of Family Social Work* (The Haworth Social Work Practice Press, an imprint of The Haworth Press, Inc.) Vol. 5, No. 3, 2001, pp. 63-78; and: *Child Mental Health: Exploring Systems of Care in the New Millennium* (ed: David A. Dosser, Jr. et al.) The Haworth Social Work Practice Press, an imprint of The Haworth Press, Inc., 2001, pp. 63-78. Single or multiple copies of this article are available for a fee from The Haworth Document Delivery Service [1-800-342-9678, 9:00 a.m. - 5:00 p.m. (EST). E-mail address: getinfo@haworthpress inc.com].

© 2001 by The Haworth Press, Inc. All rights reserved.

families in managing their concerns and difficulties are important considerations with SOC. Flexibility including the use of traditional and non-traditional services and resources is central to SOC philosophy and practice. In terms of resource identification and utilization, the family's spiritual beliefs and their faith community are often underutilized or overlooked. Reasons for this are described in this article, along with the advantages of and strategies for including them in SOC. *[Article copies available for a fee from The Haworth Document Delivery Service: 1-800-342-9678. E-mail address: <getinfo@haworthpressinc.com> Website: <http://www.HaworthPress.com> © 2001 by The Haworth Press, Inc. All rights reserved.]*

KEYWORDS. Spiritual beliefs, faith, systems, community, resources, mental health

System of care (SOC) philosophy and principles were developed and systems of care are designed and implemented as a way to improve the mental health services that are delivered to children and families (Stroul & Friedman, 1996). It is important for service providers (i.e., therapists, social workers, case managers, care coordinators) to help families identify and effectively use all available resources in order to best assist them in managing their mental health concerns and difficulties (Lourie, Katz-Levy, & Stroul, 1996). Central to SOC thinking and practice is flexibility including the use of traditional and non-traditional resources and services (Handron, Dosser, McCammon, & Powell, 1998; VanDenBerg & Grealish, 1996). The family's spiritual beliefs and their faith community are often underutilized or overlooked as resources by service providers, despite the fact that most family members consider spiritual beliefs and faith communities to be extremely important resources (Aponte, 1994,1999; Hodge, 2000; Walsh, 1999a; Wright, 1999). For example, in a book on SOC (*Children's Mental Health: Creating Systems of Care in a Changing Society*, Stroul, 1996a) very little attention is given to the importance of or use of spiritual resources when working with clients.

In this paper, SOC philosophy and practice are reviewed along with descriptions of individualized and wraparound services. In addition, reasons why service providers underutilize spiritual resources are described. An argument that these resources are important and consistent with SOC philosophy is offered. Advantages of and strategies for including spiritual beliefs and faith communities are presented along with clinical examples.

SYSTEM OF CARE PHILOSOPHY AND PRACTICE

A SOC is a philosophical framework for promoting a comprehensive, coordinated full range of community-based services (Powell et al., 1999). A *system* of care can be contrasted with a *continuum* of care. A *system* of care is broader in that it includes not only programs and services (a *continuum*) but also the processes and structures to ensure that services are provided in a coordinated, cohesive manner. A SOC has been defined by Stroul and Friedman (1986) as follows:

> A system of care is a comprehensive spectrum of mental health and other necessary services which are organized into a coordinated network to meet the multiple and changing needs of children and adolescents with severe emotional disturbances and their families. (p. 3)

According to Stroul and Friedman (1996), the values and principles of SOC dictate that services should be:

- Child centered and family focused
- Community based
- Well coordinated and integrated
- Focused on the child's physical, emotional, social, and educational needs
- Provided in the least restrictive, most normative environment possible (i.e., family's home, child's school, family's church)
- Individualized for each child and family

Values of Individualized Services

Traditionally children and families experiencing mental health difficulties have had to fit into existing and restricted services even if those services were not what they needed. Furthermore, service providers have assessed the child and family's needs and then offered them the extant service(s) that came closest to meeting their needs. Therefore, little attention and effort was given to tailoring the services to better meet the child and family's needs. Recently, individualizing services has been widely accepted as a basic premise for SOC. Moreover, the philosophy and values underlying individualized services are very similar to the philosophy for a SOC (Lourie, Katz-Levy, & Stroul, 1996). There are four values that are especially significant for individualizing services: partnership with families, cultural competence, strengths-based, ecological orientation, and unconditional care. Each of these values plays an important role in promoting individualized services and in designing and implementing systems of care for each family.

The first value in individualizing services is partnership with families. Toward this end, family members should be full and complete partners in every aspect of service delivery (Friesen & Huff, 1996; Koroloff, Friesen, Reilly, & Rinkin, 1996; Osher, defur, Nava, Spencer, & Toth-Dennis, 1999).

Families should play a role in assessment, service design, service delivery, and evaluation of services. This goal of partnership with families presents challenges and opportunities for service providers and families.

The second value is cultural competence. Services should be offered that are sensitive and responsive to cultural, racial, and ethnic differences (Lourie, Katz-Levy, & Stroul, 1996; Stroul & Friedman, 1996). The child and family's culture, race, and ethnicity should be considered in all phases of treatment planning and delivery, and the cultural, ethnic, and racial makeup of the group of providers should reflect this consideration. According to Stroul and Friedman (1996), "The implementation of this value requires careful attention to such factors as location of services, culturally sensitive assessments, emphasis on the family, staffing patterns, training, and use of natural helpers" (p. 5).

It is not possible to provide culturally sensitive services in a traditional fashion. Benjamin and Isaacs-Shockley (1996) stated, "Cultural competence involves working in conjunction with natural, informal support and helping networks with the minority community (e.g., neighborhood organizations, churches, spiritual leaders, healers, and community leaders)" (p. 476). Further, these researchers believed that the strength and effectiveness of services depended upon the provider's knowledge of and ability to mobilize these informal networks and natural support systems for their clients.

Third, instead of focusing exclusively on problems and pathology during assessment, attention is given to identifying the family's strengths and maintaining an ecological orientation. An ecological orientation is more than just being aware of teachers, neighbors, therapists, physicians, and ministers in a community. An ecological orientation promotes a sense of wholeness and teamwork in the lives of families. Traditionally, when someone in a family experiences severe emotional disturbances a number of services invade the family's life. This invasion is usually not welcomed by the family and each service's purpose becomes defeated because of the lack in connection between them.

Although many services may be available to families, the network that connects all of the resources is non-existent, and therefore leaves families feeling more frustrated. Unfortunately, the family's frustration may be perceived by professionals as resistance to treatment; however it may be that the client perceived counter messages from service providers who had different goals for the family. On behalf of the service providers, this orientation may be very difficult to digest for some professionals who do not see themselves as systemic or do not typically work with others when helping families. In working under a SOC philosophy, service providers are not asked to change their field of work only to enhance their service by including a network of providers and significant others when working with families. This teamwork is truly ecological when multiple resources are utilized and when service providers and other significant persons join together with the family to create and work toward a family goal.

Attention to the family's strengths and their ecology creates opportunities for service providers and family members to notice solution possibilities and increases the hope in both. It is important to identify strengths and to build upon them in treatment planning and service delivery. Also, it is important to identify resources and sources of support in the family's ecology that can be used to address the family's concerns and difficulties.

The fourth value, unconditional care, is especially challenging to uphold. Unconditional care means that services should be available to all families ("no reject") and that once connected to a service a family will be maintained in treatment ("no eject") (Dennis, 1997). This commitment obligates providers to do "whatever it takes" to ensure that the child and family receive clinically appropriate services in the least restrictive setting. If crises and changing needs occur, providers can then reconfigure services rather than dismissing the child and family or referring them elsewhere (Lourie, Katz-Levy, and Stroul, 1996). This value puts a large responsibility on providers to be creative and flexible in their thinking and practice.

Process of Individualized Services

Lourie, Katz-Levy, and Stroul (1996) stated that in addition to the four values, "The process of individualizing services includes four major features: interagency collaboration; case management/care coordination; wraparound services, including an array of traditional and nontraditional services; and flexibility of funding and services" (p. 434). These features are what make it possible for providers to work in partnership with families to individualize their services. Without interagency collaboration, care coordination, flexibility of funding and services, and access to and use of wraparound services, it is not possible to tailor services to meet the needs of children and families or to reconfigure those services as crises and changing needs are encountered. Ensuring that these major features are met puts a greater expectation of accountability on providers and administrators.

The first feature, interagency collaboration, extends from the ecological orientation by promoting a sense of team within and between agencies who provide multiple services. Once again, interagency collaboration extends beyond interdisciplinary care to include a system of care that supports a multi-service connection with the family and creates a succinct goal established by the SOC and the family.

The second feature, case management/care coordination is needed as well to ensure that service providers are advocating for the family's needs and that all team members are working together with the family towards a common goal. Case managers also make sure that all necessary services are being utilized and reassesses when new services should be added (Stroul, 1996b).

Behar (1986) first coined the term wraparound services, the third feature, when presenting a rationale for providing flexible dollars to pay for nontraditional services. Currently, the concept of wraparound services is applied broadly to connote the creative combination of all types of services, resources, and supports that are needed by a child and family (Lourie, Katz-Levy, & Stroul, 1996). The wraparound process is more than a new service plan; it is a philosophy of child- and family-driven service provision (Dollard, Evans, Lubrecht, & Schaeffer, 1994). Furthermore, wraparound is emerging as an alternative to the traditional treatment planning processes inherent in categorical services for children and families (VanDenBerg & Grealish, 1996).

The willingness to engage in developing non-traditional, flexible services in concert with traditional services such as psychotherapy is the means to achieving wraparound (Handron, Dosser, McCammon, & Powell, 1998). Working with wraparound services requires providers and family members to think beyond the typical and routine service delivery to embrace the creative and nontraditional. The goal is to create an individualized, intensive, and comprehensive service plan that allows the child and family to stay together and in their home community. In other words, it is doing whatever is necessary in collaboration with the family to meet their needs. As such, the wraparound approach enriches a SOC and thereby increases its capacity to help children and families (Lourie, Katz-Levy, & Stroul, 1996).

The fourth feature is flexibility of funding and services. The flexibility of funding follows a concept whereby money is attached to a family for the purchase of services and not to a program for the delivery of services (Burchard & Clark, 1990). This creativity in funding allows for flexibility in services by supporting increases or decreases in services and in changes in types of services when needed.

SOC AND SPIRITUAL RESOURCES

The effectiveness of a SOC depends upon the ability of providers to access individualized, flexible, and wraparound services. To develop and utilize these types of services, providers must draw upon all available resources for children and families–formal and informal, traditional and nontraditional. It can easily be seen that designing and implementing a system of care in a community is an awesome challenge, as is putting in place the individualized and wraparound services to meet the needs of each unique family. Upholding the values described above requires a paradigm shift for providers, administrators, and family members. This is clearly not "business as usual." Perhaps the biggest difference between SOC thinking and practice and "business as usual" is the attention to identifying and using nontraditional resources and services. Two of the most significant and influential resources could be the family's spiritual beliefs and their faith communities. The use of spiritual resources fits well with SOC values and principles. However, these resources are often underutilized or overlooked when providing services to children and families even within the framework of a SOC. Given the demands and challenges of providers who work with children and families coping with serious emotional difficulties, it is important to include all available resources especially those most important to the family.

SPIRITUAL RESOURCES

Although religious, philosophical, and spiritual values are acknowledged as important in understanding families (Carter & McGoldrick, 1998), until recently little has been written on using faith as a resource when providing mental health services to families. In addition, most service providers received little, if any, training in assessing, understanding, using a client's spiritual beliefs or faith, or in collaborating with the clergy (Weaver, Koenig, & Larson, 1997). There are several possible reasons for the exclusion of spiritual beliefs and faith when providing services to families.

The most likely reason for exclusion has been the separation of the scientific from unscientific. Cox (1996) stated that scientific training encourages an individual to question all knowledge and ways of viewing reality in hopes that new ideas, theories, and solutions to human problems can be found, and therefore any source of knowledge should be approached with skepticism. In contrast, Cox stated that religious leaders ask their converts to accept their truth as a matter of faith. Prest and Keller (1993) argued that service providers' quest for scientific status and credibility led to a separation from non-scientific, spiritual constructs. To be scientific means that the objective should be emphasized and subjective content should be minimized. Therefore, "spirituality" is associated with the subjective and cannot be operationalized or quantified in an objective way.

Furthermore, in an effort to be value free, service providers drew rigid boundaries between spiritual beliefs or practices and psychotherapy (Walsh, 1999b). Training for professional providers that stressed a stance of neutrality and the importance of remaining objective and unbiased tended to reinforce these boundaries. In the midst of these influences there has been a growing recognition that service providers cannot be neutral. Walsh (1999b) concluded:

> Inescapably, the practice of providing services involves the interaction of providers' and clients' value systems. Just as other aspects of culture

> (such as ethnicity, social class, and gender) influence client and provider constructions of norms, problems, and solutions, so too does the spiritual dimension of experience. What we ask and pursue–or do not–influences the therapeutic relationship, course, and outcome. We best respect our clients not by avoiding discussion of spirituality altogether but by demonstrating active interest in exploring and understanding their values and practices. It is most crucial to understand constraining beliefs and to affirm those that foster well-being. (p. 30)

So the cautions and prohibitions against including spiritual beliefs and resources in treatment of mental health concerns and difficulties have somewhat diminished.

Recently, the idea that a person's faith is a positive resource for service providers has gained acceptance. Steere (1997) and Moules (2000) discussed how postmodern ideas permit an interface between psychotherapeutic and spiritual practices. Contrary to previous writings, the argument has been made that spirituality is an important resource to use in assisting people manage and cope with problems (e.g., Anderson & Worthen, 1997; Hudson, 1998; Weaver et al., 1997). The growing interest in spirituality by family therapists and other mental health professionals is evidenced by recent appearances in the family therapy literature (e.g., *Spiritual Resources in Family Therapy* edited by Walsh, 1999c and five articles in the April 2000 issue of the *Journal of Marital and Family Therapy* in a special section entitled "Spirituality and Family Therapy").

These recent contributions to the literature promote the use of spiritual resources in the treatment of mental health concerns and offer suggestions for including spiritual resources in service delivery. Specific tools for bringing spiritual resources into psychotherapy include the spiritual genogram (Frame, 2000) and the spiritual ecomap (Hodge, 2000). There is also information on using spiritual resources with specific populations (e.g., families contending with chronic illness [Wright, 1999], families contending with trauma [Barrett, 1999], families contending with poverty [Aponte, 1999], African American families [Boyd-Franklin & Lockwood, 1999], and Latino families [Falicov, 1999]).

All of these ideas and tools can be used in designing and implementing treatment plans with children and families coping with serious emotional problems. These ideas, tools, and spiritual resources in general can be a significant component of the SOC, contributing greatly to the ability of families to meet their needs. The use of spiritual resources can supplement and complement the traditional resources that are typically included in treatment plans, thereby strengthening the plans. With families that possess a strong spiritual orientation, faith communities and spiritual leaders can become key allies in the service delivery process (Benjamin & Isaacs-Shockley,

1996). Churches and other religious institutions can also be used as sites for service delivery and training.

CLINICAL EXAMPLES

To expand on these ideas and to demonstrate the importance of spiritual beliefs and faith communities, some clinical examples will be presented. Introducing faith questions has been useful when treatment becomes "stuck." When little progress is evidenced, the service provider reviews goals, suggestions, and tasks assigned. In addition, the provider and family attempt to identify other available resources, including faith.

> KS was a 31-year-old divorced mother who had a six-year-old son in a residential treatment facility. While meeting with the therapist, KS appeared sad, discouraged, and alone in caring for her son and four-year-old daughter. The therapy session had many pauses and both therapist and KS showed little energy. To change the direction of the conversation, the observing therapy team phoned into the therapist with the directive to explore faith as a resource. When asked if faith has helped her in facing problems, KS said "yes." When asked to elaborate, KS shared how she prayed, read her Bible, and found attending church as strengthening. KS became more talkative and engaged in a lively conversation about how her current difficulties "hid" her faith until now. At the end of the session, KS verbalized more hope about her situation and left expressing confidence of how she would overcome her worries.

A mental health clinician was counseling a young adult who experienced ritualistic abuse that occurred in a religious setting. Although the clinician had a strong faith, she began having concerns about dealing with spiritual issues that were emerging in treatment. During her supervision, it was suggested the clinician contact a minister for assistance.

> KL was a 22-year-old woman who was self-referred. KL reported she was abused in a religious cult. KL was not currently attending a church, did not have a minister, and had significant concerns about her relationship with God. KL met the criteria for a dissociative disorder.
>
> During six months of outpatient individual therapy, it became apparent that mental health issues were woven together with spiritual issues. The therapist consulted with her supervisor and a minister was identified as a resource. KL was told about the availability of a minister who could assist with the therapy. For several weeks KL considered allowing the minister to take part in therapy. Upon KL's agreement, the

> minister was contacted and immediately indicated he would be willing to meet with the therapist and KL together to discuss care needs.
>
> A collaborative team approach resulted in which the minister provided counseling, clarification, and encouragement to KL while the therapist addressed her history and current functioning. Specifically, the minister prayed for and with KL. Sessions would begin and end with prayer. The minister gave KL scriptural references from the Bible and provided ministerial guidance. The therapist assessed and addressed issues that fit with the therapy goals.
>
> Once teamwork was established, the working contract was for all sessions to include both the minister and the therapist. Collaboration also occurred with a psychiatrist while KL received an antidepressant. KL completed treatment, was functioning well, and left with a good prognosis. Follow-up monitoring eighteen months after discharge indicated she continued to function well, to have a strong, Christian faith, and to live a stable, productive life.

Throughout KL's therapy process, the therapist noted the importance of a therapy team that provided on-going monitoring and discussion of treatment progress. Also, the therapist made audiotapes of sessions that were reviewed during her supervision. Finally, the therapist networked with a medical school resource–a dissociative disorders study group for staff development. The therapist and minister met periodically to review this collaborative approach, to assess interventions and the evolving treatment plan, and to unify efforts. The minister also used his support group to process his experiences during the treatment process.

A final clinical example of positive use of faith and spirituality will demonstrate the importance of maintaining flexibility so that services can be set up when needed to best meet the needs of clients.

> When reviewing her caseload, a therapist noted that she had several female clients with chronic anxiety and depression and who had received psychiatric care for several years. In addition, during their individual therapy sessions, each woman shared how she used faith in managing depression and anxiety. Therefore, the therapist approached each woman about creating and joining a solution-focused faith based group. The therapist and clients worked out ground rules for the group and ideas about structure, such as when and how long to meet for each session, how long the group should stay together, and when and how new members should be added. In the group meetings, the therapist assumed a collaborative, non-expert, non-hierarchical stance. She shared her experiences and personal challenges and how she drew on her faith. Still, the therapist kept focused on her role to facilitate the

group and to encourage the members to work on their personal goals. When specific spiritual issues or questions arose, the therapist referred the client to a minister or pastor. As part of this group process, it became obvious that group members were underutilizing community resources. Frequently, group members had cut themselves off from community activities including church. This led to a goal for most members to reconnect with these community resources, and they often became involved in their church fellowship.

These clinical examples show the importance of spiritual resources in the treatment of mental health concerns and difficulties. In each example, the therapist or provider team reached out to include non-traditional resources and services. For each client, the services were individualized to meet his/her specific history and needs. These examples uphold the values of considering cultural, ethnic, and racial differences, partnership, collaboration, and flexibility. In fact, the use of spiritual resources by the treatment providers expanded the treatment beyond a traditional frame to one that more closely matched the SOC philosophy.

Unfortunately, there are also examples of when faith has not been appropriately used with clients. One particular example occurred in the home of Mary and her son, Bill.

An in-home family preservation worker, who also happened to be a minister at a local church, visited Mary and Bill. The minister had asked questions about the family's issues and also had asked about Mary's marital status. Mary mentioned that she was separated but the relationship with her husband was heading toward divorce. The family preservation worker replied that divorce is a sin and that the child needed a father. Mary continued to share information about her relationship with her husband and described incidents of domestic violence. Once again the worker stated his opinion that divorce is a sin and that the child needed a father. The focus then shifted to Bill's aggression, oppositional behaviors, depression, and suicidal ideations. The worker asked if Bill was currently on any medications. Mary responded that he was on an anti-depressant and Ritalin for ADHD. The worker then stated that he was against giving the child medication and that he would work with her to get Bill off of the medications within 10 days. The worker added that Bill was demon possessed, not mentally ill and a spiritual exorcism was needed to rid Bill of the demons. Mary was greatly offended by the worker's comments and that he had shared these stories of the demons in the presence of her children. Mary shared her spiritual background and beliefs with the worker and stated that what he had said was inappropriate. The worker concluded the session by stating that she too needed to get some help.

This example demonstrates how spirituality and faith should be included in a way that is consistent with the client's beliefs. (This of course assumes that the therapist has explored what the client's beliefs are.) Spirituality and faith when shared with clients should not be done in a way to convert clients or make clients feel inadequate or uncomfortable. The following are recommendations to consider when using spirituality in an appropriate and helpful way.

RECOMMENDATIONS

Currently, it appears that the psychotherapy field is receptive to using spiritual beliefs and faith to help people manage problems and significant personal and family issues. Articles promoting this are appearing in professional publications, and presentations are being made at professional conferences and workshops. Service providers are recognizing the need for developing approaches to work with faith and spiritual issues, feeling a lack of connection to families who are spiritual, or believe that a client may be spiritually wounded. To be helpful to persons seeking treatment, mental health professionals need to understand the role of faith and spirituality in the treatment process. The authors of this article, as did Prest and Keller (1993), think that family therapy, with its emphasis on multiple levels of interaction and context, is well suited for addressing spiritual issues. Based on our experiences and in keeping with SOC philosophy, the following recommendations are given to assist providers in including spiritual beliefs and faith communities in the design and delivery of services.

1. Reflect on your own personal faith–where it stands. It may be helpful for you to reflect on your own spiritual genogram prior to working with others. The stance of service providers is not necessarily to share our beliefs but to utilize the beliefs of the family. Therefore, the non-spiritual provider can still utilize the faith-based resources of the family. The provider's stance is one of curiosity, validation, and acknowledgement.
2. Reflect on how you were informed to think about faith, religion and providing services. Does your training and approach give you permission to explore faith or does it discourage such pursuits?
3. Seek out colleagues for consultation who acknowledge and use faith-based interventions.
4. Establish supervisory support–not only clinical but also administrative. Talk about spirituality and faith with administrators and supervisors.

5. Practice openly, not covertly or behind closed doors. Acknowledge and declare to others what you are doing.
6. Establish collaborative relationships with clergy. It may be helpful to do conjoint sessions with ministers or spiritual leaders. Also there may be times or situations that are more appropriately served by a minister.
7. Become well acquainted with clergy resources in the community. Kollar (1997) stated that consultation with pastors is crucial for maintaining professional accountability by realizing how spirituality and faith communities can be a resource in individual and family's lives.
8. Be guided by the goals of the family.
9. Explore and discuss the person's faith with respect. Attempt to learn and understand the person's spiritual life.
10. When considering how to appropriately address spiritual concerns, you should request consent to speak by telephone to a member of the clergy, with whom the client is connected.

CONCLUSIONS

Finally, in summarizing what is effective in efficient successful treatment, Duncan, Hubble, and Miller (1997) pointed out the importance of establishing hope and of revitalization. They highlighted the importance of acknowledging, exploring, and validating the person's experiences. A major resource for many individuals is faith. By drawing on this resource, the provider can validate an important aspect of the person's experience. Like the pastor, each provider should walk with the client as he/she discovers new ways of managing life's challenges.

Although some practitioners imagine that specific therapeutic techniques are the determining factor contributing to outcome, the research literature does not support this assertion. Assay and Lambert (1999) highlighted evidence-based research that suggests outcome is determined more by the person and outside extratherapeutic events than by the therapist and intervention techniques. Person and extratherapeutic factors include the individual's and family's strengths and environmental supportive elements. Included in these extratherapeutic factors are the person's spiritual beliefs and faith community.

SOC encourages a collaborative dialogue with the person, family, and community. Included in this dialogue should be "faith talk." By engaging in "faith talk" the service provider can draw on an individual's faith and religious community, and acknowledge, confirm, and validate an important aspect of the person's experience. Also, the provider may encourage the individual to rediscover and reconnect to spiritual beliefs and their faith community. Introducing faith may generate creative discoveries, innovative solutions, and new ways of managing life's challenges.

REFERENCES

Anderson, D. A., & Worthen, D. (1997). Exploring a fourth dimension: Spirituality as a resource for the couple therapist. *Journal of Marital and Family Therapy, 23*, 3-12.

Aponte, H. J. (1994). *Bread and spirit: Therapy with the new poor.* New York: W. W. Norton & Company, Inc.

Aponte, H. J. (1999). The stresses of poverty and the comfort of spirituality. In F. Walsh (Ed.), *Spiritual resources in family therapy* (pp.76-89). New York: The Guilford Press.

Assay, T. P., & Lambert, M. J. (1999). The empirical case for the common factors in therapy: Quantitative findings. In M. A. Hubble, B. L. Duncan, & S. D. Miller (Eds.). *The heart and soul of change: What works in therapy.* Washington, DC: American Psychological Association, pp. 23-25.

Barrett, M. J. (1999). Healing from trauma: The quest for spirituality. In F. Walsh (Ed.), *Spiritual resources in family therapy* (pp. 193-208). New York: The Guilford Press.

Behar, L. (1986, May-June). A state model for child mental health services: The North Carolina Experience. *Children Today*, 16-21.

Benjamin, M. P., & Isaacs-Shockley, M. (1996). Culturally competent service approaches. In B. A. Stroul (Ed.), *Children's mental health: Creating systems of care in a changing society* (pp. 475-492). Baltimore: Paul H. Brookes Publishing Co.

Boyd-Franklin, N., & Lockwood, T. W. (1999). Spirituality and religion: Implications for psychotherapy with African American clients and families. In F. Walsh (Ed.), *Spiritual resources in family therapy* (pp. 90-103). New York: The Guilford Press.

Burchard, J. D. & Clarke, R. T. (1990). The role of individualized care in a service delivery system for children and adolescents with severely maladjusted behavior. *Journal of Mental Health Administration, 17*, 48-60.

Carter, B., & McGoldrick, M. (Eds.). (1998). *The expanded family life cycle: Individual, family, and social perspectives* (3rd ed.). Boston: Allyn and Bacon.

Dennis, K. (1997). *Wraparound process.* Presentation at the annual conference of the North Carolina Family Based Services Association, Greenville, NC.

Dollard, N., Evans, M. E., Lubrecht, J., & Schaeffer, D. (1994). The use of flexible service dollars in rural community-based programs for children with serious emotional disturbances and their families. *Journal of Emotional and Behavioral Disorders, 2*(2), 117-125.

Duncan, B. L., Hubble, M. A., & Miller, S. D. (1997). *Psychotherapy with impossible cases: Efficient and effective treatment of therapy veterans.* New York: The Guilford Press.

Falicov, C. J. (1999). Religion and spiritual folk traditions in immigrant families: Therapeutic resources with Latinos. In F. Walsh (Ed.), *Spiritual resources in family therapy* (pp. 104-120). New York: The Guilford Press.

Frame, M. W. (2000). The spiritual genogram in family therapy. *Journal of Marital and Family Therapy, 26*, 211-216.

Friesen, B. J., & Huff, B. (1996). Family perspectives on systems of care. In B. A.

Stroul (Ed.), *Children's mental health: Creating systems of care in a changing society* (pp. 41-68). Baltimore: Paul H. Brookes Publishing Co.

Handron, D. S., Dosser, D. A., Jr., McCammon, S. L., & Powell, J. Y. (1998). "Wraparound"–The wave of the future: Theoretical and professional practice implications for children and families with complex needs. *Journal of Family Nursing, 4*, 65-86.

Hodge, D. R. (2000). Spiritual ecomaps: A new diagrammatic tool for assessing marital and family spirituality. *Journal of Marital and Family Therapy, 26*, 217-228.

Hudson, P. (1998, April/May). Spirituality: A growing resource. *Family Therapy News*, 10-11.

Koroloff, N. M., Friesen, B. J., Reilly, L. & Rinkin, J. (1996). The role of family members in systems of care. In B. A. Stroul (Ed.), *Children's mental health: Creating systems of care in a changing society* (pp. 409-428). Baltimore: Paul H. Brookes Publishing Co.

Lourie, I. S., Katz-Levy, J., & Stroul, B. A. (1996). Individualized services in a system of care. In B. A. Stroul (Ed.), *Children's mental health: Creating systems of care in a changing society* (pp. 429-452). Baltimore: Paul H. Brooks Publishing Co.

Moules, N. J. (2000). Postmodernism and the sacred: Reclaiming connection in our greater-than-human worlds. *Journal of Marital and Family Therapy, 26*, 229-240.

Osher, T., defur, E., Nava, C., Spencer, S., & Toth-Dennis, D. (1999). Family as faculty. In *Systems of care: Promising practices in children's mental health, 1998 Series, Vol. 1. New roles for families in systems of care* (pp. 39-62). Washington, DC: Center for Effective Collaboration and Practice, American Institutes for Research.

Powell, J., Dosser, D. A., Jr., Handron, D., McCammon, S., Temkin, M., & Kaufman, M. (1999). Challenges of interdisciplinary collaboration: A faculty consortium's initial attempts to model collaborative practice. *Journal of Community Practice, 6*(2), 27-48.

Prest, L. A., & Keller, J. F. (1993). Spirituality and family therapy: Spiritual beliefs, myths, and metaphors. *Journal of Marital and Family Therapy, 19*, 137-148.

Steere, D. A. (1997). *Spiritual presence in psychotherapy: A guide for caregivers.* New York: Brunner/Mazel, Inc.

Stroul, B. A. (Ed.). (1996a). *Children's mental health: Creating systems of care in a changing society.* Baltimore: Paul H. Brooks Publishing Co.

Stroul, B.A. (1996b). Service coordination in systems of care. In B. A. Stroul (Ed.), *Children's mental health: Creating systems of care in a changing society* (pp. 265-280). Baltimore: Paul H. Brooks Publishing Co.

Stroul, B. A., & Friedman, R. M. (1986). *A system of care for children with severe emotional disturbances.* Washington: CASSP Technical Assistance Center for Child Health and Mental Health Policy, Georgetown University.

Stroul, B. A., & Friedman, R. M. (1996). The system of care concept and philosophy. In B. A. Stroul (Ed.), *Children's mental health: Creating systems of care in a changing society* (pp. 3-21). Baltimore: Paul H. Brooks Publishing Co.

VanDenBerg, J. E., & Grealish, E. M. (1996). Individualized services and supports through the wraparound process: Philosophy and procedures. *Journal of Child and Family Studies*, *5*(1), 7-21.

Walsh, F. (1999a). Religion and spirituality: Wellsprings for healing and resilience. In F. Walsh (Ed.), *Spiritual resources in family therapy* (pp. 3-27). New York: The Guilford Press.

Walsh, F. (1999b). Opening family therapy to spirituality. In F. Walsh (Ed.), *Spiritual resources in family therapy* (pp. 28-58). New York: The Guilford Press.

Walsh, F. (Ed.). (1999c). *Spiritual resources in family therapy.* New York: The Guilford Press.

Weaver, A. J., Koenig, H. G., & Larson, D. B. (1997). Marriage and family therapists and the clergy: A need for clinical collaboration, training, and research. *Journal of Marital and Family Therapy*, *23*, 13-25.

Wright, L. M. (1999). Spirituality, suffering, and beliefs: The soul of healing with families. In F. Walsh (Ed.), *Spiritual resources in family therapy* (pp. 61-75). New York: The Guilford Press.

Service Learning and Systems of Care: Teaching Students to Learn from Clients

John H. Pierpont, PhD
Richard Pozzuto, PhD
John Y. Powell, PhD

SUMMARY. This article concerns itself with the integration of policy and practice in the professional training of Master's level social workers. The implications of policy for practice are explored and the approach of service learning is articulated as a method of linking policy and practice. This occurs within a qualitative evaluation of a System of Care (SOC) program. Students are advised to learn from their clients in order to become both better service providers and advocates. The political role of social work is also highlighted. Results of the evaluation are

John H. Pierpont and Richard Pozzuto are Assistant Professors and John Y. Powell is Professor Emeritus, School of Social Work and Criminal Justice Studies, East Carolina University.

Address correspondence to: John H. Pierpont, 216A Ragsdale Hall, School of Social Work and Criminal Justice Studies, Greenville, NC 27858-4353 (E-mail: pierpontj@mail.ecu.edu).

Appreciation is expressed to Ms. Traci Lynch for assistance in manuscript preparation.

Preparation of the manuscript was funded in part through a contract with the North Carolina Division of Mental Health, Developmental Disabilities and Substance Abuse Services, Child and Family Services, as a component of the System of Care: Training and Curriculum Development Project, funded by a grant from the Center for Mental Health Services.

Portions of this paper were presented at the 13th Annual Research and Training Conference in Children's Mental Health, Clearwater Beach, Florida, on March 6, 2000.

[Haworth co-indexing entry note]: "Service Learning and Systems of Care: Teaching Students to Learn from Clients." Pierpont, John H., Richard Pozzuto, and John Y. Powell. Co-published simultaneously in *Journal of Family Social Work* (The Haworth Social Work Practice Press, an imprint of The Haworth Press, Inc.) Vol. 5, No. 3, 2001, pp. 79-93; and: *Child Mental Health: Exploring Systems of Care in the New Millennium* (ed: David A. Dosser, Jr. et al.) The Haworth Social Work Practice Press, an imprint of The Haworth Press, Inc., 2001, pp. 79-93. Single or multiple copies of this article are available for a fee from The Haworth Document Delivery Service [1-800-342-9678, 9:00 a.m. - 5:00 p.m. (EST). E-mail address: getinfo@haworthpressinc.com].

© 2001 by The Haworth Press, Inc. All rights reserved.

included. *[Article copies available for a fee from The Haworth Document Delivery Service: 1-800-342-9678. E-mail address: <getinfo@haworthpressinc.com> Website: <http://www.HaworthPress.com> © 2001 by The Haworth Press, Inc. All rights reserved.]*

KEYWORDS. Service learning, empowerment research, learning from clients, strengths-based practice

INTRODUCTION

Typical of the social work profession generally, social work graduate students most often choose to focus on direct, clinical practice over other practice areas such as policy and administration. Further, they often fail to see the connections between direct practice and social policy (Powell & Causby, 1994). Gordon (1994) stated that students generally see policy courses as "peripheral" to their interests. This disregard for policy has serious implications for students in social work and other professional training programs as well as for their clients. First, this failure to appreciate the significant impact public policies make on recipients of social services prevents students from using policy as a means of helping clients ameliorate their problems. Second, it allows students, who soon become professionals, to view client complaints about social programs as little more than another client problem or deficit, rather than learning from clients about the inadequacies of policies and their implementation as social programs. Finally, social policy–its critique, development, and implementation–is an important venue for achieving, and for teaching students about, social justice. The failure to appreciate the role of policy in practice, the impact of policies on clients' lives, and the first-hand knowledge clients have of policy, prevents students from working to overturn ineffective or unjust policies and from viewing clients as expert resources on policies and programs that need to be changed or abolished.

Although most students do not enter social work with an interest in politics or policy (Wolk, Pray, Weismiller, & Dempsey, 1996), practicing social work requires the assumption of certain policy roles (Gordon, 1994; Jansson, 1999; Wyers, 1991). Wyers (1991) suggested that direct service practitioners "must understand and analyze the effect of extant social policy on clients and participate in the modification of social policy that is harmful to clients and in the elimination of policy deficits by working for new policy" (p. 246). Given the importance of policy to the practice of social work and students' general lack interest, the task for social work educators is formidable.

Rocha (2000) suggested that *service learning* is an appropriate and useful method for teaching social policy. According to Rocha, service learning is a type of experiential learning that enables students to participate in an activity that serves their community and at the same time encourages them to reach a deeper understanding of course content by reflecting on their community service. According to Bringle and Hatcher (1996) this approach heightens civic responsibility and political participation. A service learning approach can be found across a variety of disciplines including political science (Barber & Battistoni, 1993), social work (Leeds, 1996), and English (Novak & Goodman, 1997).

STRATEGY FOR LINKING PRACTICE AND POLICY

In order to (a) facilitate students' recognition of the inseparability of practice and policy, and (b) assist students' discovery of the invaluable resource of client experience and feedback, the authors gave students a service learning assignment related to the evaluation of a multi-county child mental health pilot project. The pilot project established an interdisciplinary, collaborative System of Care (SOC) program to better meet the needs of children with severe emotional disturbances and their families. The anticipated benefits of the service learning project were many, e.g., to demonstrate for students the direct impact public policies have on the well-being of clients; to enrich students' understanding of and appreciation for the importance of including clients (and family members) in developing policy and evaluating policy implementation in practice; to enable students to experience first-hand the connections between social policy; professional practice, and social justice; and to provide a service to the community *vis à vis* evaluation of a local SOC, child mental health program.

With the growing popularity of the strengths perspective in social work practice, much has been said in recent years regarding the importance of learning from clients and of viewing clients as experts on their capabilities, needs, and deficits (Saleeby, 1997). However, the authors are unaware of any attempts to avail students of clients' expertise for the express purpose of demonstrating the direct connections between practice and policy and the effects of policy for good and ill on clients. The tasks associated with this assignment provided a context in which students learned directly from clients about the impact of a social policy and how that policy could be improved and better implemented. By relying on clients as the primary source of data for the evaluation project, students also experienced first-hand clients' expertise in evaluating policies and in assessing collaborative, interdisciplinary practice.

THE SERVICE LEARNING PROJECT

In a course for advanced Master of Social Work (MSW) students specializing in child and family services, the authors developed a service learning project in which the 18 students in the course evaluated the SOC program using qualitative research methods. Each student was assigned to interview two people from a sample of participants representing three groups: (1) families, (2) service providers, and (3) administrators, planners, or consultants. Students wrote summaries of their interviews independently and later formed groups to perform content analyses on the collected data. Results of the content analyses were written up, given to their professors, and discussed in class. Finally, students conducted a community forum to share their findings. At the conclusion of the forum, students completed a brief survey to help evaluate the effectiveness of the service-learning project as a learning experience.

Students were asked to use interviews to learn from participants about the relative success or failure of a collaborative project that was intended to "revolutionize" service delivery. Specifically, students were to ascertain (a) what participants would do differently as a group and individually if the project were starting anew; and (b) how well System of Care core values and guiding principles (see table in Stroul, B., & Friedman, R. (1986)). *A system of care for children and youth with severe emotional disturbances* (rev. ed., p. 17). Washington, DC: Georgetown University Child Development Center, National Technical Assistance Center for Children's Mental Health) were maintained from the viewpoints of the three informant groups. Again, the intended benefits included students' learning about the impact of policy on clients, for good and ill; and the value of including clients in developing and implementing public policy. Student recognition of societal inequities and a commitment to advocate for clients or continue to work with the agency are viewed as additional and welcome benefits.

The importance of obtaining information for program evaluation from persons associated with service delivery programs, e.g., direct practitioners, supervisors, and agency administrators, is rather self-evident for students. However, obtaining and evaluating information from clients represents new learning, even though one of the purposes of research is to provide information for clients as well as for professionals (Holmes, 1992). The authors drafted the SOC service learning assignment with the intent of drawing from clients' expertise. Therefore, this evaluation project is compatible with what is known as "empowerment research" (Rappaport, 1990). Empowerment research furthers the search for knowledge while also allowing research informants to speak for themselves and to address their own needs (Rappaport, 1990). Empowerment research "not only allows for participation by subjects, but relies upon and solicits it" (Holmes, 1992, p. 159). Whereas participants in this System of Care research project were from three distinct groups (families; service providers; and administrators, planners, and consultants), all of the participants were viewed equally as experts. All of the participants, therefore, were asked to give their views pertaining to the relative success or failure, strengths and limitations, of the program. They were also asked for recommendations that might improve the program in the future.

After all interviews were completed, MSW students were randomly assigned to one of three content analysis groups corresponding to the three cohort groups that were interviewed. Each student read all the interviews for his or her cohort group, and then individually recorded the major themes and unusual responses that he or she observed. Later students met in groups and, through a consensus process, developed a joint content analysis of the data. Six students served on the Family Interviews Content Analysis group for the family interviews. The following is a summary of a family interview. The interviewee is a parent who received services through the SOC program and who later became a family advocate. Personal information has been deleted or altered to protect the confidentiality of the interviewee. Headings in the interview narrative correspond to topics addressed on the interview form.

FAMILY INTERVIEW SUMMARY

Understanding of the System of Care

> At first I didn't understand what System of Care was, nor why we were involved, until 1997 when my daughter began receiving services. When we did start receiving services, the first thing that was a service to me was the family advocate, because I felt no one else in the world could feel the way I did or know the things I was going through. Attending the support meetings gave me an awareness of services and was therapy to me, to be able to work and talk with other parents. If I had known that all the services we received were available, before she got worse, maybe they could have helped prevent that. Most parents still don't know what System of Care means. As a parent advocate, I found that once the people involved found that I was also a parent, it opened a new avenue for relationships with that person.

Involvement

> My daughter was introduced to System of Care, in 1995, but didn't receive services until 1997, because she was a level 3. She eventually became a level 2, which meant that she got worse, instead of better. Once my daughter attempted suicide and was hospitalized, they sent me some forms. Mental Health put me in touch with a parent advocate who actually introduced me to the System of Care process.

Evaluation

Strengths

It strengthened me as a parent and an advocate for my own child. It gave an awareness of her illness. System of Care is potentially a good program. I don't know what it started out to be, I only can tell you what the end was for me. The only problem I had with System of Care was keeping a case manager. We have had 4 case managers since 1997.

Challenges

The real challenge was to try to get more families involved. Parents have so many other things going on in their lives, that it is hard for them to take the time to do things for one child, when all the children in the home have issues. When we have support meetings there was no place to put the children and transportation was also a large problem. I was very fortunate to have only one child, therefore, my time and energy went to getting services for her, even then I didn't get every service I needed. I think this was probably due to the fact that it was impossible for every professional to attend every meeting. Just trying to get them all together was a challenge. Another problem was getting the children to really trust the therapist and talk with them. I personally have always wanted to have a support meeting for the children, to come together in a forum and ask questions if need be, to show children that the professionals are not their enemies, they are there to help. The only way to trust someone is to socialize with that person so that a relationship is built.

Replication

Personally I would not keep one agency in charge of the purse, because whoever holds the purse strings, holds the control and power. It should be equally shared and should include family members on a board, set up to handle decisions. The family member is the only one who really knows what that child needs. Needs should be discussed with the parents, we also need to listen to what the child feels, he or she needs. During the last year and a half of System of Care, it really began to work.

Starting Anew

I would have liked for them to treat us as their equals and not to look down at us because we don't cross every "t" and dot every "i." I would like for them to listen to me, they are in control of my child's life. These are our children and we see them just as you see your own child.

Child-Centered and Family Focused Value

The child can't be helped unless the family is helped, because even if the child is sent away, eventually that child will come back home. All families are functional and have their strengths. If a child sees that something is helping their family they are more apt to go along with it. I would like to see more in-home visits, and more things that are family driven.

Community Based Value

The community needs to be more involved, and that includes the faith community, businesses, and the police. Some of the things that need to be done could have been accomplished with community support. Night therapists would also help, because so many of the parents work during the day.

Seamless Array of Services Value

A child's emotional state touches every one of their physical, social and emotional needs. My daughter has a problem with re-entry into school. If she is sick, it is a problem for her to go back. Her emotions actually made her physically sick. System of Care offered a lot of services, but getting everyone together was almost impossible, yet all-important to helping the child. The value of that is priceless. As a parent, if I could go to a meeting where there was no one pointing a finger, where people were only there to come up with a plan, that would be great. *(Interviewee asked that interviewer put a star by the last sentence, noting its importance.)

Cultural Competence Value

I believe that cultural competence starts at home, everyone is different. To be competent we must find out what goes on in each home and respect that. Remember a family may want to pray before a meeting. If so, honor it–honor their culture.

The above summary is representative of the family interviews insofar as each interview provides a family member's perspective on significant aspects of the SOC program, including the project's strengths, challenges to participating in the program, suggestions for improving the program, etc. Again, in the SOC program, family members are considered experts with regard to their families, their needs, and their experience of service delivery programs. Their perspective is crucial if planners, administrators, and direct service practitioners are to learn from existing SOC programs.

STUDENT EVALUATION OF THE SERVICE LEARNING ASSIGNMENT

A brief survey instrument was administered to each student at the end of the project just prior to the community forum. Students were asked to respond to these statements: "The assignment helped me integrate some of what I learned in practice class with policy"; "The assignment helped me better understand how policy affects clients"; "The assignment helped me better understand how clients can contribute to formulating better policy and programs." Students were asked to assign a number 5 through 0, to each question where 5 = Strongly Agree, 4 = Agree, 3 = Not Sure, 2 = Disagree, 1 = Strongly Disagree, 0 = No Opinion. To the first question, "The assignment helped me integrate some of what I learned in practice classes with policy," six students strongly agreed, five students agreed, two students were not sure, and five students did not answer the question. To the question "The assignment helped me better understand how policy affects clients," ten students strongly agreed and eight students agreed. To the question "The assignment helped me better understand how clients can contribute to formulating better policy and programs," seven students strongly agreed, ten students agreed, and one student was not sure. Responses to the questions are presented in the Appendix.

Students were also asked to respond to two open-ended statements: "The most helpful aspect of the assignment was . . . ," and "The least helpful aspect of the assignment was . . . " Responses to the first question fell into two general categories pertaining to "meeting or learning from program participants," and "learning about policy and program," respectively. Eight responses suggested that experiences such as "gaining a better understanding of how important clients could be in developing policy," "actually meeting the participants," and "hearing from program participants" were the most useful aspect of the service learning assignment. Four responses indicated that experiences such as "learning systems of care," "learning both the strengths and weaknesses of the program," and "seeing different perspectives of how administrators knew what was going on versus how the families view the services they are receiving" were the most helpful aspect of the assignment. Other responses indicated that analyzing data, learning interviewing techniques, and learning to formulate an evaluation was also helpful.

Responses to the statement "The least helpful aspect of the assignment was . . . " generally pertained to assignment logistics such as time frame for different aspects of the assignment and difficulty contacting informants. Overall, students' assessments of the service learning assignment were quite positive insofar as they seemed to reflect significant learning in the areas anticipated by the assignment.

CONCLUSIONS

The authors have drawn three significant conclusions from the service learning project assignment. First, service learning assignments can be useful in teaching students the value of listening to clients to obtain information regarding the effects of policy. Second, through service learning, students may learn experientially that, although practice and policy may be distinguished one from the other, they cannot be separated in practice. Finally, the service learning assignment served the community by providing valuable information about the program to its program planners, administrators, and direct practitioners, and perhaps more importantly, by eliciting information from program participants that may be used to improve existing and future policies and their implementation.

A useful extension of this and similar service learning assignments might include follow-up studies, at various points in time, to ascertain whether students applied knowledge gained from this assignment once they became practicing professionals. For example, it would be instructive to know whether students are using lessons learned from the service learning assignment to advocate for policy and program changes on behalf of client groups such as children with serious emotional disturbances and their families. Bringle and Hatcher (1996) found that service learning assignments heighten students' civic responsibility and political participation. A question of interest would be whether students who helped to carry out this project become involved in advocacy efforts, at any level, for societal improvement and social justice. Finally, it would be useful to know whether students who have participated in service learning assignments such as the one described here practice from a client-centered, strengths-based approach, i.e., whether they view clients as important sources of knowledge and expertise. If students do become professionals who practice from a strengths-based perspective, was the service learning assignment a significant factor in their decision to do so?

Recipients of social services have much to teach professionals and students, and it appears that service learning may be an effective means of educating professionals and students alike. Clearly, service learning warrants additional study to better gauge its effectiveness in conveying the importance of consulting with clients about policies and programs; demonstrating the inseparability of policy and practice; and providing useful community service.

REFERENCES

Barber, B. R., & Battistoni, R. (1993). A season of service: Introducing service learning into the liberal arts curriculum. *PS: Political Science and Politics, 26*, 235-240.

Bringle, R. G., & Hatcher, J. A. (1996). Implementing service learning in higher education. *Journal of Higher Education, 67*(2), 221-239.

Gordon E. B. (1994). Promoting the relevance of policy to practice: Using the ADA to teach social policy. *Journal of Teaching in Social Work, 19*(2), 165-176.

Holmes, G. (1992). Social work research and the empowerment paradigm. In D. Saleeby (Ed.), *The strengths perspective in social work practice.* New York: Longman.

Jansson, B. (1999). *Becoming an Effective Policy Advocate.* Pacific Grove, CA: Brooks/Cole.

Leeds, J. (1996). Training student volunteers for community service: A model of collaboration. *Journal of Community Practice, 3*(2), 95-102.

Novak, C. C., & Goodman, L. J. (1997). Safer contact zones: The call of service learning. *The Writing Instructor, 16*(2), 65-77.

Powell, J. Y., & Causby, V. D. (1994). From the classroom to the Capital–from MSW students to advocated: Learning by doing. *Journal of Teaching in Social Work, 9*(1/2), 141-154.

Rappaport, J. (1990). Research methods and the empowerment social agenda. In P. Tolan, C. Keys, F. Chertok, and L. Janson (Eds.), *Researching Community Psychology.* Washington, DC: American Psychological Association.

Rocha, C. (2000). Evaluating experiential teaching methods in a policy practice course: The case for service learning to increase political participation. *Journal of Social Work Education, 36*(1), 53-64.

Saleeby, D. (1997). *The strengths perspective in social work practice.* New York: Longman.

Wolk, J., Pray, J., Weismiller, T., & Dempsey, D. (1996). Political practica: Educating social work students for policy making. *Journal of Social Work Education, 32,* 91-100.

Wyers, N. (1991). Policy-practice in social work: Models and issues. *Journal of Social Work Education, 27*(3), 241-250.

APPENDIX

Content Analysis–Families Cohort

Item #1–Their Understanding of System of Care

A. Student's judgment of each interviewee's understanding

1.	Limited	3	2	4	0	2	2	= 13
2.	Moderate	5	3	2	5	2	2	= 21
3.	Good	1	4	3	4	5	5	= 20

B. The common theme which emerged

1. The program was for children with special needs
2. The program provided a source of support for the parents of children with special needs
3. The program put families in touch with needed services
4. The program provided a collaborative effort between helping professionals and families in need

C. The unusual comments or inconsistencies were

1. Parents were not aware of all the services available to them
2. Some parents thought System of Care was a person
3. One parent will miss System of Care's services (the idea was for the services to continue)

Item #2–How Involvement with System of Care Started

A. Common themes

1. Referral from Mental Health or some other service provider
2. Referral from System of Care advocate

B. Unusual comments or inconsistencies

1. Child behavior had to get worse before the child could be referred

Item #3–Evaluation of System of Care from the Parent's Perspective

A. Strengths

1. The parent/child focus was strong
2. It was a strengths based program
3. Case managers were really involved
4. Communication style was good, things were presented in an understandable form
5. There was an attempt made to be culturally competent

APPENDIX (continued)

Unusual comments and inconsistencies

1. Communication was sometimes a problem
2. Some of the parents felt that they were looked down upon

B. Challenges and Problems

1. One problem expressed was that case mangers were hard to keep
2. Some felt that the focus was on money and not on families and children
3. It was also difficult to pull everyone together at one time
4. There were turf and control issues
5. More families should have been involved earlier

Unusual comments and inconsistencies

1. One parent said that there were no problems or challenges
2. Some felt that transportation was an issue, but some said they were provided ample transportation

C. Problems with policy or program

1. System of Care was great concept, it looked good on paper, but it was hard to put into reality
2. Some of the parents had difficulties with one agency holding the funding

D. Extent to which the program was effective at meeting the needs and addressing problems

1. System of Care provided a forum for professionals and parents to collaborate
2. The program helped parents to gain a better understanding
3. System of Care helped parents gain a better understanding of their child's needs and diagnosis
4. Some parents felt empowered by their experience with System of Care, while others felt like they were a part of the process

Item #4–Advice for Replication of System of Care

A. The things parents felt should be kept are

1. Federal level: keeping the lines of communication open was important to some parents
2. State level: It was suggested that things be left as they are, "it's working"
3. Local: Parents felt that the principles and values needed to be kept, as well as family and board meeting and the parenting classes–One parent felt that WE CARE was very useful

B. Things which need to be changed on any level

1. Federal: Parents want more involvement–More funding is another thing that parent's feel needs to be done
2. State: Parents felt like the money should not be held by any one person or agency
3. Local: Parents feel that more people should have involvement earlier

Unusual comments or inconsistencies are

1. Parents feel they should be aware of funding allocations

C. Things which need to be deleted

1. "Cut out the fussing" about money

D. Things recommended for adding

1. The parents wish to see more involvement by the faith community
2. It was also felt that the community needs to be aware of System of Care

Unusual comments

1. One parent commented that System of Care didn't take them to dinner often

Item #5–Personal Changes if System of Care was Starting Anew

A. Common themes were

1. Parents felt they would be more talkative
2. Some thought they would attend more meetings
3. Others felt they would advocate and encourage more parents to get involved
4. Some hoped to be treated as equal partners
5. Some wished the community could be involved earlier

B. Unusual comments or inconsistencies were

1. Parent would be more assertive as an advocate

APPENDIX (continued)

Item #6–Review of the System of Care Principles and Values

A. Child-centered and family focused–with needs of the child and family dictating the type and mix of services provided

1. The principles focused on child strengths
2. The child and their family was the main focus
3. The family was given a voice
4. There was positive communication between parents

Unusual comments or inconsistencies were

1. Some parents felt that communication was good, some did not
2. Others felt that not every case manager focused on the family

B. Community based with management and decision making at the community level

1. Parents felt more community involvement was needed

Unusual comments were

1. Some felt that the community did not even know what System of Care was

C. Comprehensive, seamless array of services that addressed the child's physical, emotional, and educational needs

1. Parents felt it was difficult to get everyone together at one time for a meeting

Unusual comments and inconsistencies

1. About half of the parents stated that it was a seamless array of services and the other half felt that it was not

D. Culturally Competent program and services that honored and respected cultural, racial and ethnic differences

1. No apparent themes were found here

Unusual comments and inconsistencies

1. Some felt that work was needed in this area
2. Some thought that there was some racial tension
3. One parent mentioned that it did not serve the Spanish speaking population
4. Others felt that more education was needed in this area
5. Some felt that the program was culturally competent

Item #7–Other Thoughts or Suggestions for System of Care

A. Some of the parents felt that they needed to keep the program because it was helpful

Unusual comments or inconsistencies were

1. Some felt that every graduate should be taught the System of Care, not just at the graduate level
2. One parent remarked about the fact that System of Care had been like a big family discussing problems
3. Others felt the program should continue, under another name

APPENDIX 2

Results of the Student Evaluation of the Service Learning Assignment

5 = Strongly Agree, 4 = Agree, 3 = Not Sure, 2 = Disagree, 1 = Strongly Disagree, 0 = No Opinion

	5 SA	4 A	3 NS	2 D	1 SD	0 NO
1. The assignment helped me integrate some of what I learned in practice class with policy.	6	5	2			5
2. The assignment helped me better understand how policy affects clients.	10	8				
3. The assignment helped me better understand how clients can contribute to formulating better policy and programs.	7	10	1			

The Complexities of Implementing a Wraparound Approach to Service Provision: A View from the Field

Kaye McGinty, MD
Susan L. McCammon, PhD
Valerie Poindexter Koeppen, MA

SUMMARY. The authors offer the perspective of several service providers on the benefits and barriers encountered in implementing the wraparound model within the context of a federally funded project to enhance a local system of care. The Pitt Edgecombe Nash–Public Academic Liaison project was instituted in three rural counties in Eastern North Carolina. A hallmark of this program was the role of families as

---

Kaye McGinty is Assistant Professor, Department of Psychiatric Medicine, Body School of Medicine and Susan L. McCammon is Professor, Department of Psychology, East Carolina University. Valerie Poindexter Koeppen is a licensed Psychological Associate in Greenville, NC.

Address correspondence to: Kaye McGinty, Department of Psychiatric Medicine, East Carolina University School of Medicine, 600 Moye Boulevard, Brody 4E, Greenville, NC 27858-4354 (E-mail: kmcginty@mail.ecu.edu).

Appreciation is expressed to Ms. Traci Lynch for assistance in manuscript preparation.

Preparation of the manuscript was funded in part through a contract with the North Carolina Division of Mental Health, Developmental Disabilities and Substance Abuse Services, Child and Family Services, as a component of the System of Care: Training and Curriculum Development Project, funded by a grant from the Center for Mental Health Services.

[Haworth co-indexing entry note]: "The Complexities of Implementing a Wraparound Approach to Service Provision: A View from the Field." McGinty, Kaye, Susan L. McCammon, and Valerie Poindexter Koeppen. Co-published simultaneously in *Journal of Family Social Work* (The Haworth Social Work Practice Press, an imprint of The Haworth Press, Inc.) Vol. 5, No. 3, 2001, pp. 95-110; and: *Child Mental Health: Exploring Systems of Care in the New Millennium* (ed: David A. Dosser, Jr. et al.) The Haworth Social Work Practice Press, an imprint of The Haworth Press, Inc., 2001, pp. 95-110. Single or multiple copies of this article are available for a fee from The Haworth Document Delivery Service [1-800-342-9678, 9:00 a.m. - 5:00 p.m. (EST). E-mail address: getinfo@haworth pressinc.com].

© 2001 by The Haworth Press, Inc. All rights reserved.

treatment partners with the emphasis on collaboration among agencies, families and service providers. The actual process is organized by a service coordinator and led by an individual service team. While implementing the wraparound model, benefits and barriers were encountered at all levels of intervention. The authors suggest that quality-monitoring efforts should include the task of assessing implementation on an ongoing basis with an emphasis on analysis of the barriers and benefits encountered and subsequent midstream corrections to improve the wraparound model for each individual community. *[Article copies available for a fee from The Haworth Document Delivery Service: 1-800-342-9678. E-mail address: <getinfo@haworthpressinc.com> Website: <http://www.HaworthPress.com> © 2001 by The Haworth Press, Inc. All rights reserved.]*

KEYWORDS. Wraparound model, systems of care, quality improvement

Over the past twenty years the needs of children and adolescents with serious emotional disturbances (SED) and their families have become a focus of many new treatment efforts. Various projects to develop local systems of care and promote extensive family involvement, interagency collaboration and expansion of needed services have been undertaken (Stroul & Friedman, 1996). A widely used approach to service delivery within the system of care model is the wraparound process (Rosenblatt, 1996). The wraparound process is not a program or service, but a process that is used to help communities develop individualized plans of care for children with SED. Each individualized plan is developed by a child and family team that helps design, implement and monitor the interventions. Various authors (MacFarquhar, Dowrick, & Risley, 1993; VanDenBerg & Grealish, 1996) have documented the importance of all services being coordinated in order for the multiple needs of SED youth and their families to be met appropriately and effectively.

In the wraparound planning process, significant persons involved in the child's life come together to create a plan that addresses various life domains and focuses on the strengths of the child and family. VanDenBerg and Grealish (1996) described the key components of the process: convening a team with the child, family, traditional service providers and nontraditional members (such as extended family, friends, clergy, mentors and community members); keeping a family perspective of the needs; developing supports and services around the individual's needs and strengths; incorporating interventions into one plan; and making a commitment to the process. Furthermore, there is an emphasis on keeping the child in his/her home community and ensuring that services are provided in a culturally competent manner. Since these children are served by multiple agencies, the importance of collaboration is emphasized and evaluation methods are implemented to monitor the outcomes of the process.

The concept of providing wraparound care makes an appealing package, as Rosenblatt (1996) observed. He offered a simple metaphor, "wraparound services are one of the most attractive packages for children with multi-system needs" ("ribbons and bows") (p. 113-114). However, he elaborated that it is the "twine and tape" of careful definition, refinement, implementation, and research that help this practice package withstand the tough handling of use in the field. To wrap the wraparound package with tape and twine will require interpretation and understanding of negative findings, as well as celebration of successes and positive results.

Clark, Prange, Stewart, McDonald, and Boyd (1998) characterized the body of wraparound initiative research literature as offering growing, but limited, support for the superiority of such individualized approaches for serving children with the severest emotional and behavioral problems and their families. That the levels of clinical improvement observed do not show the magnitude of effect we would hope for is not surprising, given that "the field is still defining and refining the wraparound process and children's systems-of-care strategies" (p. 536). They suggested that it is difficult to achieve the intensity of intervention needed to serve children and families with complex, multisystem needs, to adequately match the needs with services, and to ensure the fidelity of adherence to the wraparound intervention approach.

Our objective is to offer an integrated perspective of several service providers (a psychiatrist, a psychologist, and a service coordinator) on the challenges to the strength and integrity of implementing the wraparound model within the context of a federally funded project to enhance a local system of care. We hope that examples from our community will be useful to illustrate the benefits and difficulties in faithfully implementing the wraparound model. In addition, we offer insights into the complexity of operationalizing wraparound principles and recommendations for addressing the barriers.

THE WRAPAROUND PROCESS IN THE PEN-PAL PROJECT

The actual process of implementing wraparound in a community setting was part of the PEN-PAL (Pitt Edgecombe Nash–Public Academic Liaison) project. This project was one of the Center for Mental Health Services (CMHS) sites as part of the Child and Adolescent Service System Program. It was instituted in three rural counties in Eastern North Carolina. The respective 1994 populations were 56,811 (Edgecombe County), 82,788 (Nash County), and 116,088 (Pitt County). According to the 1993 Children's Index (NC Child Advocacy Institute, 1993), all three counties had a substantial need for improved services. These communities had a significantly greater number of teen parents, children living in poverty, and numbers receiving aid to families with dependent children relative to the state average. The median family income, high school graduation rate and Scholastic Aptitude Test (SAT) scores, useful in predicting successful outcomes during the first year of college, were well below North Carolina averages. Furthermore, juvenile and violent arrests were almost three times the state average, and children in out-of-home placements were two times that of the state average. The three counties are served by two area mental health programs, three school districts, three health departments, three departments of social services, two judicial districts, and a state university. The area mental health programs administered and coordinated the project among the agencies, with support from staff of the Child and Family Services Section of the North Carolina Division of Mental Health, Developmental Disabilities and Substance Abuse Services.

The overriding goal of the project was to reduce out of home placements for children with the presence of a *Diagnostic and Statistical Manual, Fourth Edition* (DSM IV) (APA, 1994) Axis I diagnosis as a major inclusion criterion. A hallmark of this project was the role of the families as treatment partners with the emphasis on collaboration among agencies, families and service providers. Service Coordinators (case managers) were responsible for organizing and maintaining this collaborative process. The organizing event at the child/family level was the Individual Service Team (IST) (in some sites, called the Child and Family Team) meeting whereby treatment planning evolved with the participation of relevant persons to the family and child.

In implementing individualized service approaches, the case manager plays an essential role and has been described as the "backbone" of the system of care (Katz-Leavy, Lourie, Stroul, & Zeigler-Dendy, 1992). The main role of the service coordinator is to help mobilize resources to meet the needs of the child and family. In order to accomplish this goal, there are a core set of functions, including assessment, service planning, service implementation, service coordination, monitoring and advocacy. Some of the service coordinators also served in the role of therapist as well.

In PEN-PAL the service coordinator began by establishing contact with the child and family with a focus on developing rapport and emphasizing the significance of the family's input in the process. Information was presented using various available formats (verbal and written) to promote understanding. The concepts of strengths based evaluation and treatment were explained (VanDenBerg & Grealish, 1996). In order to encourage family participation, the service coordinator asked questions to determine the important people in the life of the family and child. This process was essential to begin helping the family identify potential members for their IST. These individuals could include both child service workers (teachers, social workers, etc.) and other community agents (friends, family, clergy, community leaders) important to the family. As the discussion progressed to the strengths and needs of the child, the service coordinator might make suggestions to the family if needed, especially since the families were often accustomed to negative assessments of their child's situation. Then, an inventory of the family's supports and resources was undertaken in more depth for the family to further develop a list of key people in their life including family members, friends, neighbors, church members and community contacts. Once the family was able to complete this process, potential team members were contacted and an IST was formed. The meeting place and time for the IST meeting were negotiated with the family and team. Frequently chosen sites included the mental health center, the school, or the family's home. Before the first meeting it was important for the service coordinator to assure that forms for sharing information and a comprehensive confidentiality form were completed by all members of the team.

A family's initial IST meeting began with introductions and an explanation of how each participant was involved with the child and family. Confidentiality was stressed and reviewed. The service coordinator led the group in developing guidelines for group functioning. Some commonly endorsed group guidelines included confidentiality, contributing information in a timely manner, respecting others, keeping the child and family focus, maintaining the strengths based approach, and time limited meetings (about 1 hour). The service coordinator continued with an overview of the IST process, including an emphasis on the strengths based approach. Throughout this process the service coordinator encouraged the family to participate and promoted the family's agenda. The IST members identified the strengths of the child and family from their individual perspectives. This is an important step to gain different perspectives from those who know the child and family in various contexts. Once this was completed, the needs of the child and family were discussed. Both strengths and needs were viewed in the context of life domains. Major life domain areas included safety, housing, family, social life, education and vocational training, medical, psychological and emotional, and legal needs (VanDenBerg, 1993). Then, interventions and supports were proposed to address the needs of the child and family and the team prioritized the most critical needs in order to promote successful outcomes. Finally, team members identified tasks to complete, and the next meeting date was arranged.

As the wraparound process progressed, the IST identified various strengths and needs of the child and family and attempted to identify interventions that would address these needs. The service coordinator worked closely with the family to access appropriate services. Flexibility in service provision was emphasized which may have included providing transportation to attend appointments or providing certain services in the home. Also, some interventions required creativity and foresight in the use of both traditional services and nontraditional community resources in multiple steps.

The service coordinator in this type of system became a community broker who must work at all levels of the community and system hierarchy. The first step was to attempt to find donated community services or time to meet nontraditional needs. However, if donated services were not available, it became critical to be able to access monies for interventions or parts of interventions that are out of the "traditional mental health arena." These types of interventions can be imperative to help a child overcome a major hurdle. Behar (1986) outlined a rationale for using "flexible" dollars to pay for nontraditional services to help SED children remain in the community and participate in traditional service programs. Flexible funds were tapped as a last resort and were used creatively to help barter for other resources and funds or to purchase services or items unavailable through any other means. Furthermore, the IST members were important in this phase because they often assumed various roles in promoting the successful implementation of many of the interventions, along with the child and family.

As the wraparound process continued, the service coordinator reviewed all the services the child and family received and promoted the coordination of these services. This was done at the individual and family level, as well as at the system level. Service coordination has been shown to be extremely important for promoting improved outcomes in SED children (Stroul, 1996). In the initial stages, this might require daily phone calls or meetings to refine the IST plans. The service coordinator helped to maintain the communication with IST members and the family, promoting flexibility and effectiveness of interventions. As this process continued, the frequency of formal meetings typically decreased, and informal communication with all team members was maintained by the service coordinator.

This approach represents a facilitated, participatory process whereby the child and family voice their strengths and needs. Over time the goal is for the family to take ownership for their problems and solutions along with the gathered community (IST team) (Whitbeck et al., 1993). As the process develops there is a reframing of strengths and needs tied to life domains to produce an individualized, in-depth treatment plan. The team interaction can provide an avenue for the child, family and formal/informal community agents to work together to promote the child's development and participation in the community.

BARRIERS AND BENEFITS ASSOCIATED WITH THE WRAPAROUND PROCESS

In many parts of the United States wraparound approaches have been rapidly implemented. This occurred before there had been adequate articulation of wraparound principles and operationalization of the processes and practices. This has resulted in increased challenges to accurate implementation of the model (Clark & Clarke, 1996). Barriers can exist at all levels of intervention. This is not surprising when one realizes that the successful application of the wraparound process requires shifts in multiple venues including attitudes, programming and funding (Burchard & Clarke, 1990). We will discuss implementation barriers we encountered at the child/family level, the agency level, and broader community and policy levels. In addition, possible benefits associated with using the wraparound process will be identified. Examples will be drawn from our work with "Demarcus," a 14-year-old African-American adolescent, and his IST during his eighth grade year.

Child/family level barriers and benefits. With most families we felt we were able to move from a relationship in which the family tolerated agency involvement to a family-provider partnership, or at least episodes of partnership. For example, the child and family team for Demarcus was convened early in the school year. This was in response to his first day of class, when Demarcus brushed past the teacher to leave the room, and the teacher had him charged with assault. In court, the family court judge noted the presence of several members of the wraparound team and Demarcus's grandfather. He urged Demarcus to take advantage of such a support team, and agreed to dismiss the charge if there were no further incidents. The grandfather felt that the presence of team members influenced the disposition and he expressed appreciation of the team's participation. We felt like we were partners with the family, but were reminded that building a real partnership, especially across socioeconomic, ethnic, and racial groups, does not come easily. Two of us were at the family's home one day when Demarcus's (African American) great-grandmother answered the phone and said, "I can't talk now–there's two white ladies here."

One of the greatest challenges was that of moving from family involvement to "a family-centered approach." This was complicated by the difficulty of gaining access to the real players in some of the families. In Demarcus's family, the Department of Social Services (DSS) had legal guardianship, although he was placed with his grandfather. In reality, the grandfather lived with his girlfriend and Demarcus lived with his great-grandmother in a different home outside of town where he took care of her as much as she cared for him. His siblings lived with another relative, and he was forbidden by DSS to have contact with his mother because of her ongoing drug use. However, Demarcus did have contact with her, and as soon as DSS relinquished legal custody to the grandfather, he moved in with his mother again. The complexity of working with the three-generation family, and having an "off-limits" member who really was a player but could not be acknowledged, was not something any of the professional staff was truly prepared to tackle. The ideal of having a service plan that is the family's plan, and is truly family-driven, can be more challenging than it sounds. In situations in which we were able to develop true partnerships, service plans were more practical and ecologically valid, in contrast to some of our experiences with office-based and expert-oriented models of practice.

When working with children and families, we became aware that the introduction of a new way of receiving help can be intimidating, especially for a parent of a child with severe emotional and behavioral challenges. The family may have difficulty trusting the system and its agents, although the concept of family participation is being touted. This possible barrier speaks to the need for a close relationship with the service coordinator and the IST members for the family to feel empowered and to participate fully. Perhaps we might have addressed this through greater inclusion of parent advocates to provide families with additional supports. Evans, Armstrong, and Kuppinger (1996) described the unique contribution of parent advocates as one-on-one supports to parents; while service coordinators tended to work with parents on issues of behavior management, service planning and education. The families in this study noted the importance of the assistance of both service coordinators and parent advocates. Team members were all valued and role differentiation was understood. With the help of the service coordinator, parent advocate and team the child and/or family may be able to overcome any fears or dislikes of the team experience or participatory role that the wraparound process requires.

Barriers and benefits at the child service provider and supervisor level. Many child service providers have not been educated to provide care with this model. Indeed, Hanley and Wright (1995) noted that the most serious long-term challenge for the new children's mental health paradigm is the need for a cadre of professionals who support its implementation, along with the need for graduate educational programs to address this issue. Therefore, providers may have difficulty delivering care in this manner and working with families as partners. In addition, the child service worker may not agree with the focus on the family and this attitude may lead to difficulties with implementation. Variations in performance of the service coordinators or their supervisors, and increased turnover due to stress, high case loads, lack of staff commitment, or anxiety about grant funding can also adversely affect implementation of this process.

Suggestions for what supervisors can do to define shape, and maintain norms which promote wraparound practice have been offered by Friedman and Poertner (1995). In PEN-PAL one of the service coordinators was a master's level psychologist who was required by licensing law to have weekly supervision with a doctoral level psychologist. That supervisor attempted to use the concepts of participatory and empowering supervision described by Friedman and Poertner, and emphasized helping the service coordinator clarify problem situations and brainstorm alternative actions and community resources. Since the supervising psychologist and psychiatrist were associated with a university, this brought the benefit of the university library and support resources of undergraduate and graduate students looking for practicum experiences to the aid of the service coordinator.

Another major barrier to providing this type of care is the complexity of implementing the strengths based approach. Many service coordinators and team members have commented that the strengths and needs of the child and family are fairly easy to identify. However, once you view these in the context of life domains and try to develop interventions and supports, application becomes more difficult. Our training programs have been helpful in teaching methods and instruments for identifying strengths. However, there is little training that teaches how to build on those strengths to meet needs, how to use the strengths to develop positive behavioral response repertoires, and how to use ecological and social network theory to build social networks and community supports when they are lacking. It takes creativity, imaginative problem-solving, extensive knowledge of the local community, and multiple community brokers to accomplish these tasks.

An innovative effort in Demarcus's service plan was implemented to build on his willingness to work and desire to earn some spending money. One of the service team members arranged with her church for summer funds to pay Demarcus for three hours of weekly cleaning for the church. She provided transportation and worked alongside him during the work periods. He enjoyed the opportunity to earn spending money and had an opportunity to show his good work ethic in being an industrious worker. His grandfather, a hard-working man, was pleased, and judging from an essay Demarcus wrote at school, he felt proud as well.

> I stayed focused on my work . . . I made $5.00 an hour. When I and [sic] finished with my work, I look back over it and then think I have done a good job with it. Susan liked it too and the people who go to the church like the way I clean. So they want me to go back to work at the church in the future. That makes me feel proud of my self.

In addition to the complexity of this model, the time that is required to accomplish this process is enormous and many of the IST members may have limited time to commit. Thus, the service coordinator takes on more tasks and may not have the contacts needed to accomplish these tasks. Other potentially useful participants may not be on the team. Lack of relevant skills may lead to individualized treatment plans that are poorly conceived or poorly executed.

On the other hand, the individualized service plans may be executed with care and still not be adequate. An example from Demarcus's plan was an attempt to build on his interest and skill in playing basketball to meet a recreational need. With his service coordinator's help the pervious year he had gotten on a Parks and Recreation league team, and his team won the championship. His grandfather agreed that he could sign up to play again this year. The service coordinator was able to secure flex funds to cover the cost of the necessary physical exam to allow participation, and provided transportation for the exam. But when Demarcus's grandfather took him to sign up for the league, the cost was greater than anticipated, as their address was outside the city and county residents were charged at a rate higher than his grandfather was able or prepared to pay. So they went home without registering. When the service coordinator found out what had happened the deadline for registration had passed, and no more players were being added to the league. The increased cost (few dollars) should not have been a barrier, but either the grandfather did not know that Parks and Recreation can waive a fee, or it was not acceptable to him to ask. As a result, this component of the service was not realized, despite an attempt to build on an interest and strength with the support of the service coordinator, and family.

Lack of support from coworkers and supervisors as a result of many of the aforementioned barriers may interfere with the service coordinators' successful completion of the job. Indeed, Miles and VanDenBerg (1995) have described various responses to individualized care that coworkers may express including: "we're already doing this; I wasn't hired to do this; we don't have time; we're losing control-what about clinical issues; this is really different than what we used to do; and we get to share responsibility with others." Unless all members of the organization are educated about this process, it can make it very difficult to use with families. Service coordinators have stated that having support groups and participating in staff meetings/conferences with staff trained in this model helped them deal with their isolation and provided needed support to continue learning how to work with this model. Moreover, these multidisciplinary groups allowed trainees from multiple disciplines (marriage and family therapy, nursing, psychiatry, psychology, and social work) to have an opportunity to gain insight into being a practitioner working with this type of model.

The benefit of being able to share responsibility with others was the strongest selling point of the wraparound model to staff from the various agencies. In Demarcus's situation the team especially worked at providing an exceptional amount of support to the school. The team acknowledged the very demanding situation Demarcus's special education teacher faced. He had eleven students in the class, many with significant behavior problems, and a class history of having had a student attacked and seriously injured in the class the previous year. Initially, team members were appalled at the teacher's strategy of suspending students to achieve a more manageable class size. But rather than directly confront this method, the team developed a plan for a "classroom wrap," reasoning that if the teacher had adequate support, he would not rely so heavily on suspension as a management tool. University faculty and graduate students provided volunteer support in the classroom to help Demarcus, and worked with other students as well. Materials for the teacher to use as reinforcers, academic resources, and materials for the classroom were donated, as well as consultation on behavior management. Probably the most tangible aspect of the year's work for the team was Demarcus's success in completing his grade. The teacher, social services case manager, and mental health service coordinator each appreciated sharing the professional responsibility, and the family felt supported. The university faculty and students extended their learning by spending time in the middle school environment and enjoyed the contact with the students in the class.

Community and policy level barriers and benefits. In general, community members were positive about this project and were frequently willing to be involved. Barriers to community support for the project included lack of knowledge about the concept and difficulty finding ways to promote the model in community venues. The rural setting may have contributed to these barriers. Many community leaders were very busy and involved in multiple projects and initiatives, leaving them little time to contribute to this new initiative. When a community representative did become more engaged it was usually after direct or indirect contact with one of the children and/or families who were involved in the wraparound process. For example, following the success of the "classroom-wrap," the classroom teacher, social services worker, and a mental health service coordinator successfully established an innovative plan for funding a classroom support person to assist another student with special needs in the class.

For mental health agencies the wraparound process represents a new way of providing services and requires programmatic transition that can be difficult and challenging. The support of agency administrators is vital to the success of such a change. Once the leaders determine that the wraparound process will become part of their system, their entire workforce should be included in the educational process. Hopefully, this would be conducive to fewer intra-agency barriers.

Although the wraparound approach encourages building on local resources, it is important to understand that services can be obtained occasionally, but not always, for free. At times it is possible to get reduced rates or group rates for activities or interventions. The administrators involved in the financial aspects of the organization are integral to this process, especially with the need to have flexible funds available during individualized service planning. Twenty five percent of the programs in MacFarquhar, Dowrick, and Risley's survey (1993) indicated that difficulties with flexible funding were their most significant problem. The reported problems were with acquiring adequate funding to provide individualized care as well as in the ability to use funds in a flexible manner. These multiple steps can be difficult to accomplish in a busy, human service agency. Therefore, lack of administrative or funding support can be a major barrier to successful implementation of the wraparound process.

Now that the CMHS funding is no longer supporting our local system of care, we have developed a local source of flexible funds. It is a fund called "Kids' Want Adds," based on the premise that "meeting the *wants* of kids *adds* to the community." The fund resides with the local chapter of the Mental Health Association, and is sponsored by a local bank and the newspaper. A committee of local service providers, a parent, and the Mental Health Association Director screen requests for funds, which may be submitted by any child and family serving agency. Periodically ads are published in the newspaper, describing some of the "wants," such as funds to attend a summer camp or skill-building program. Donations are accepted for the specified children or for the general fund. Community response has been positive and providers are beginning to enhance service plans by making them more comprehensive in supporting positive developmental activities for the children they serve. The establishment of this community-supported fund has been one successful strategy for bypassing some of the aforementioned organizational constraints.

Significant policy barriers can interfere in using the wraparound process. Fiscal and legal constraints (especially confidentiality), bureaucratic rigidities and differences in system mandates can all lead to obstacles in interagency collaboration (Knitzer, 1989). Difficulties matching this type of treatment approach to various agency guidelines and paperwork requirements were especially problematic for this project. Many child service agencies have enormous amounts of paperwork requirements that are already in place and they must complete these, along with anything additionally added by the wraparound process. Any additional paperwork tasks further overload these workers. In our community we have not been able to overcome this barrier.

Local and state governments have a vested interest in the improved functioning of SED children and their families, therefore, these leaders should be included in these initiatives. With competing community economic needs, political leaders will be viewing this initiative amongst many others. It is important to educate the local leaders on the wraparound process, goals, objectives and outcomes. It should be emphasized that by helping children and families, communities are strengthened. However, dealing with the political leaders and their budget office is difficult without data that can support the efficacy of this method. If the results of outcome research are not compelling, this may be a significant barrier when dealing with elected officials. If the local politicians do not accept this initiative as important to their community, there may be a lack of commitment to its success and this could ultimately interfere with the successful implementation of such a system.

Examination of the outcome data from the PEN-PAL project are encouraging in that a significant portion of the children improved, or stabilized, in the six months following their enrollment into the program, based on scores on the Child and Adolescent Functional Assessment Scale (CAFAS) (Hodges, 1990, 1994 rev.). For example, Fernandez, Behar, Diamond, O'Donnell, and Kaufman (2000) reported that in the African American male group (N = 54) the CAFAS scores six months after enrollment showed improvement for 35% of the group, while 43% remained the same. Although stabilization of functioning for a young person in distress may be a significant accomplishment, we share Friedman's (1997) concern that "it may be that without more conclusive findings there will be a decrease in funding for existing services even if the field is moving in the right direction"(p. 24).

Furthermore, given our experience with the complexities of implementing the wraparound process and maintaining the focus over time, there are concerns that deficiencies in implementation, and insufficient agency/community support for the process, affected the quality of the intervention. In fact, the degree to which client gains, or at least stabilization, in PEN-PAL were due to the wraparound process is unknown. Although quality monitoring efforts were included in the PEN-PAL project, the fidelity of implementation of the model was not assessed for all clients, and has not been linked with the outcome data.

CONCLUSIONS

In view of the barriers encountered in this service initiative, we encourage researchers, administrators, service providers, and families to pay particular attention to the task of assessing implementation on an ongoing basis, including analysis of the barriers encountered and midstream corrections to address the identified barriers. Friedman (1997) explained that this is a difficult task, "because the interventions are complex, individualized, and multifaceted and often occur at both the service and the system levels." However, tools are being developed to assist, such as the SOC Practice Review (Hernandez, in press) and efforts to assess wraparound fidelity are underway (Malysiak Bertram, Bertram Malysiak, Rudo, & Duchnowski, 2000). Malysiak Bertram et al. (p. 198) delineated three theory-based constructs essential to maintaining the integrity of the wraparound approach:

- Construct 1. Families must act as informed, decision-making participants.
- Construct 2. The teams must be well-composed and well-constructed.
- Construct 3. Together, team members must identify and use strengths in the home, school and community to meet needs that are identified across systems and life domains. The emphasis on these constructs is compatible with our observations of issues critical in application of a wraparound. Perhaps the use of such measures as these authors recommend can promote improved implementation of the wraparound model, making it more than a "pretty package," and advancing it as a powerful tool for helping to improve the outcomes for youth with serious emotional difficulties and their families.

REFERENCES

American Psychiatric Association (1994). *Diagnostic and statistical manual of mental disorders*. Fourth Edition. Washington, DC: Author.

Behar, L. (1986). A state model for child mental health services: The North Carolina experience. *Children Today*, 16-21.

Burchard, J. D. & Clarke, R. T. (1990). The role of individualized care in service delivery system for children and adolescents with severely maladjusted behavior. *Journal of Mental Health Administration, 17*(1), 48-60.

Clark, H. B. & Clarke, R. T. (1996). Research on the wraparound process and individualized services for children with multi-system needs. *Journal of Child and Family Studies, 5*(1), 1-5.

Clark, H. B., Prange, B. L., Stewart, E. S., McDonald, B. B., & Boyd, L. A. (1998). An individualized wraparound process for children in foster care with emotional/behavioral disturbances: Follow-up findings and implications from a controlled study. In M. H. Epstein, K. Kutash, & A. Duchnowski (Eds.), *Outcomes for children and youth with emotional and behavioral disorders and their families: Programs and evaluation best practices* (pp. 513-542). Austin, TX: Pro-ed.

Evans, M. E., Armstrong, M. I., Kuppinger, A. D. (1996). Family-centered intensive case management: A step toward understanding individualized care. *Journal of Child & Family Studies, 5*(1), 55-65.

Fernandez, M. E., Behar, L., Diamond, J., O'Donnell, M. & Kaufman, M. (2000). NC PEN-PAL: Who got better? Who got worse? In C. Liberton, C., C. Newman, K. Kutash, & R. Friedman (Eds.), The 12th Annual Research Conference Proceedings, A System of Care for Children's Mental Health: Expanding the Research Base (February 21 to February 24, 1999) (pp. 41-43). Tampa, FL: University of South Florida, The Louis de la Parte Florida Mental Health Institute, Research and Training Center for Children's Mental Health.

Friedman, R. (1997). Services and service delivery systems for children with serious emotional disorders: Issues in assessing effectiveness. In C. T. Nixon & D. A. Northrup (Eds.), *Evaluating Mental Health Services: How Do Programs for Children "Work" in the Real World?* (pp. 16-44). Thousand Oaks, CA: Sage.

Friedman, C. R. & Poertner, J. (1995). Creating and maintaining support and structure for case managers: Issues in case management supervision. In B. J. Friesen & J. Poertner (Eds.). *From Case Management to Service Coordination for Children with Emotional, Behavioral, or Mental Disorders: Building on Family Strengths* (pp. 257-274). Baltimore: Brookes.

Hanley, J. H. & Wright, H. H. (1995). Child mental health professionals: The missing link in child mental health reform. *Journal of Child and Family Studies, 4*, 383-388.

Hernandez, M. (in press). Use of the system of care practice review in the national evaluation: Evaluating the fidelity of practice to system of care principles. *Journal of Emotional and Behavioral Disorders.*

Hodges, K. (1990, 1994 rev.). *The Child and Adolescent Functional Assessment Scale.* Ypsilanti, MI: Eastern Michigan University, Department of Psychology.

Katz-Leavy, .J, Lourie, I., Stroul, B., & Zeigler-Dendy, C. (1992). *Individualized services in a system of care.* Washington, DC: Georgetown University Child Development Center, National Technical Assistance Center for Children's Mental Health.

Knitzer, J. (1989). Children's mental health policy: Challenging the future. *Journal of Emotional & Behavioral Disorders, 1*(1), 8-16.

MacFarquhar K.W., Dowrick, P. W., & Risley, T. R. (1993). Individualizing services for seriously emotionally disturbed youth: A nationwide survey. *Administration and Policy in Mental Health, 20*(3), 165-174.

Malysiak Bertram, R., Bertram Malysiak, B., Rudo, Z. H., & Duchnowski, A. J. (2000). What maintains fidelity in a wraparound approach? How can it be measured? In C. Liberton, C. Newman, K. Kutash, & R. Friedman (Eds.), *The 12th Annual Research Conference Proceedings, A System of Care for Children's Mental Health: Expanding the Research Base* (February 21 to February 24, 1999), (pp. 197-201). Tampa, FL: University of South Florida, The Louis de la Parte Florida Mental Health Institute, Research and Training Center for Children's Mental Health.

Miles, P. & VanDenBerg, J. (1995). The PEN-PAL project: Intensive training on the wraparound process. (Unpublished document from training workshop. VanDenBerg Consulting, 9715 Bellcrest Road, Pittsburgh, PA 15237).

North Carolina Child Advocacy Institute. (1993). *Children's Index.*

Rosenblatt, A. (1996). Bows and ribbons, tape and twine: Wrapping the wraparound process for children with multi-system needs. *Journal of Child and Family Studies, 5*(1), pp. 101-107.

Stroul, B. (1996). Service coordination in systems of care. In B. A. Stroul (Ed.). *Children's Mental Health: Creating systems of care in a changing society* (pp. 265-280). Baltimore, MD: Brookes.

Stroul, B. A. & Friedman, R. M. (1996). The system of care concept and philosophy. In B. A. Stroul (Ed.). *Children's Mental Health: Creating systems of care in a changing society* (pp. 3-21). Baltimore, MD: Brookes.

VanDenBerg, J. E. & Grealish E. M. (1996). Individualized services and supports through the wraparound process: Philosophy and procedures. *Journal of Child and Family Studies, 5*, 7-21.

VanDenBerg, J. E. (1993). Integration of individualized mental health services into the system of care for children and adolescents. *Administration & Policy in Mental Health, 20*(4), 247-257.

Whitbeck, J. Kimball, G., Olsen, D., Lonner, T., McKenna, M. & Robinson, R. (1993). *An analysis of the interaction among systems, services and individualized and tailored care: A report from the field.* Olympia, WA: Washington Division of Mental Health.

Index

© 2001 by The Haworth Press, Inc. All rights reserved.

For Product Safety Concerns and Information please contact our EU representative GPSR@taylorandfrancis.com Taylor & Francis Verlag GmbH, Kaufingerstraße 24, 80331 München, Germany

Printed and bound by CPI Group (UK) Ltd, Croydon, CR0 4YY

08/06/2025

01897011-0004